WM 18 PAT

D1141625

MRCPsych Papers 1 and 2

600 EMIs

MRCPsych Papers 1 and 2

600 EMIs

Ashok G Patel MBBS DPM FRCPsych
Consultant General Adult Psychiatrist (Retired)
South Essex Partnership University NHS Foundation Trust
Luton, UK

Samir Shah MBBS MRCPsych MSc
Consultant Psychiatrist in General Adult Psychiatry
Cheshire and Wirral Partnership NHS Foundation Trust
Macclesfield, UK

Gursharan Lal Kashyap MBBS, DCH, MD, MRCPsych
Specialist Registrar Year 5 in Psychiatry
South Essex Partnership University NHS Foundation Trust
Bedford Hospital
Bedford, UK

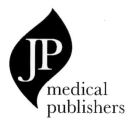

JP
medical
publishers

London • Philadelphia • Panama City • New Delhi

© 2014 JP Medical Ltd.
Published by JP Medical Ltd,
83 Victoria Street, London, SW1H 0HW, UK
Tel: +44 (0)20 3170 8910
Fax: +44 (0)20 3008 6180
Email: info@jpmedpub.com
Web: www.jpmedpub.com

The rights of Ashok G Patel, Samir Shah and Gursharan Lal Kashyap to be identified as the editors of this work have been asserted by them in accordance with the Copyright, Designs and Patents Act 1988.

All rights reserved. No part of this publication may be reproduced, stored or transmitted in any form or by any means, electronic, mechanical, photocopying, recording or otherwise, except as permitted by the UK Copyright, Designs and Patents Act 1988, without the prior permission in writing of the publishers. Permissions may be sought directly from JP Medical Ltd at the address printed above.

All brand names and product names used in this book are trade names, service marks, trademarks or registered trademarks of their respective owners. The publisher is not associated with any product or vendor mentioned in this book.

Medical knowledge and practice change constantly. This book is designed to provide accurate, authoritative information about the subject matter in question. However readers are advised to check the most current information available on procedures included and check information from the manufacturer of each product to be administered, to verify the recommended dose, formula, method and duration of administration, adverse effects and contraindications. It is the responsibility of the practitioner to take all appropriate safety precautions. Neither the publisher nor the editors assume any liability for any injury and/or damage to persons or property arising from or related to use of material in this book.

This book is sold on the understanding that the publisher is not engaged in providing professional medical services. If such advice or services are required, the services of a competent medical professional should be sought.

Every effort has been made where necessary to contact holders of copyright to obtain permission to reproduce copyright material. If any have been inadvertently overlooked, the publisher will be pleased to make the necessary arrangements at the first opportunity.

ISBN: 978-1-907816-41-3

British Library Cataloguing in Publication Data
A catalogue record for this book is available from the British Library

Library of Congress Cataloging in Publication Data
A catalog record for this book is available from the Library of Congress

JP Medical Ltd is a subsidiary of Jaypee Brothers Medical Publishers (P) Ltd, New Delhi, India

Commissioning Editor: Steffan Clements
Design: Designers Collective Ltd

Typeset, printed and bound in India.

Preface

The MRCPsych examinations are extremely challenging, and candidates must be meticulous in their preparation if they are to stand any chance of success. Understanding this principle has been fundamental during our preparation of this book, and we have endeavoured to provide sufficient EMI revision material for each element of the curriculum. We are confident that by using this book, readers will be well armed to face the EMI component of the Paper 1 and 2 exams.

The book is organised into two sections, the first focusing on the MRCPsych Paper 1, the second on the MRCPsych Paper 2. In order to facilitate revision, the first four chapters in each section are mapped to the respective curriculum. The final chapter in each section is left intentionally unstructured, thereby providing two mock exams, representative of the EMI component of the Paper 1 and 2 exams, which readers can use to practise under exam conditions. All questions are based on the curriculum and thorough answers have been provided to explain the rationale behind each correct answer option.

The burden of editorship has been wisely spread to harness varied expertise. In psychiatry, innovation in practice tends to be evolutionary rather than revolutionary, and much of our knowledge remains to be translated into practical innovations in patient care. It is our intention that this book will help psychiatry trainees not only to pass the MRCPsych examination, but also to improve their patient care. We believe that the book will assist trainees, trainers, educational and clinical supervisors, College tutors, Directors of Medical Education, SAS tutors and Training Programme Directors in preparation for the MRCPsych examinations.

Ashok G Patel
Samir Shah
Gursharan Lal Kashyap
December 2013

Contents

Acknowledgements

We would like to thank the colleagues and friends who have helped us as we prepared this book. They have been a great source of useful advice and suggestions and have read the draft papers to make sure that the questions and answers were compatible with the MRCPsych Paper 1 and 2 exams.

We are also most grateful to the many people behind the scenes without whose help this book would not have been possible. In particular, we would like to thank the publishers, especially Steffan Clements, Hannah Applin and Katrina Rimmer for their encouragement and support from the very beginning to the end of the project. Special thanks go to Sue Keely and Mrs Vasanthi Varadharajan in preparing the manuscripts.

We would like to thank Nicola Cowdery, Deepak Garg, Vineel Reddy, Khurram Sadiq, Ajaya Upadhyaya, Dinesh Khanna, Faisal Pervez, Sanjith Kamath, Vishelle Kamath, Basavaraja Papanna and Juhi Mishra for their support and encouragement.

Finally, we would also like to thank the families of the authors and our own families for putting up with us as inevitably the book has been written during evenings, weekends and holidays.

AP, SS, GK

Contributing Authors

Syed Ashraf MBBS PGCHM
Chapters 1 & 6: Questions and Answers
Specialty Doctor in Psychiatry
South Essex Partnership University NHS
Foundation Trust
Bedford Hospital
Bedford, UK

Gursharan Lal Kashyap MBBS DCH MD
MRCPsych
Chapters 1, 5 & 7: Questions and Answers
Specialist Registrar Year 5 in Psychiatry
South Essex Partnership University NHS
Foundation Trust
Bedford Hospital
Bedford, UK

Vishelle Kamath MBBS MRCPsych
Chapters 2 & 7: Questions and Answers
Consultant Old Age Psychiatrist
South Essex Partnership University NHS
Foundation Trust
Houghton Regis, UK

Komal A Patel BSc MBChB MRCS
Chapters 2, 5, 6 & 10: Questions and Answers
Core Trainee Year 2 in Surgery
Surrey & Sussex Healthcare NHS Trust
East Surrey Hospital
Redhill, UK

Roshelle Ramkisson MBBS MRCPsych
MSC (Health and Public Leadership) PGDip
Psychiatry MDCH
Chapters 3 & 8: Questions and Answers
Consultant Psychiatrist in Child and Adolescent
Psychiatry
Pennine Care NHS Foundation Trust
Royal Oldham Hospital
Oldham, UK

Madhavan Seshadri MBBS DPM MRCPsych
Chapters 3 & 9: Questions and Answers
Specialist Registrar Year 6 in Psychiatry
South Essex Partnership University NHS
Foundation Trust
Bedford Hospital
Bedford, UK

Samir Shah MBBS MRCPsych MSc
Chapters 4 & 9: Questions and Answers
Consultant Psychiatrist in General Adult
Psychiatry
Cheshire and Wirral Partnership NHS
Foundation Trust
Macclesfield, UK

Raman Sharma MBBS MSc (Psychiatric Practice)
MRCPsych
Chapters 4, 8 & 10: Questions and Answers
Specialty Doctor in Psychiatry
South Essex Partnership University NHS
Foundation Trust
Bedford Hospital
Bedford, UK

Section 1

MRCPsych Paper 1 EMIs

Chapter 1

Test questions: 1

Questions: EMIs

HISTORY AND MENTAL STATE EXAMINATION

Theme: Sleep disorders

Options for questions: 1–3

A	Advanced sleep phase syndrome	E	Non–24-hour sleep-wake disorder
B	Circadian rhythm disorder not otherwise specified	F	Rhythmic movement disorder
		G	Shift-work sleep disorder
C	Hypersomnia	H	Sleep drunkenness
D	Irregular sleep–wake pattern		

For each of the following cases, select the single most likely sleep disorder. Each option may be used once, more than once or not at all.

1. A 37-year-old man works in an office, and complains of early sleep onset (e.g. 6–8 pm) and early morning wakening.

2. A 41-year-old man exhibits stereotyped repetitive movements of the head and neck, occurring immediately before sleep, which are sustained into light sleep.

3. A 39-year-old man has a sleep–wake period of more than 24 hours, which leads to a steady pattern of daily delays in sleep onset and wake times by 1–2 hours.

Theme: Interviewing skills

Options for questions: 4–6

A	Closed questions	D	Open question
B	Introductory statement	E	Polythematic questioning
C	Normalising statement	F	Reflection

For each of the following cases, select the single most appropriate interviewing skill. Each option may be used once, more than once or not at all.

4. Are you feeling depressed for no apparent reason?

5. It is not uncommon for people in your situation to feel so low when things are bad.

6. Tell me, why are you here? What can I do for you? Did you see your doctor before coming here?

COGNITIVE ASSESSMENT

Theme: Publications on cognitive assessment

Options for questions: 7–9

A   Berg (1948)
B   Eysenck and Eysenck (1975)
C   Folstein et al (1975)
D   Hathaway and McKiney (1983)

E   Luria (1966)
F   Rey (1964)
G   Rorschach (1921)
H   Wechsler (1987)

For each of the following cognitive function tests, select the single most likely associated publication. Each option may be used once, more than once or not at all.

7. A test for measuring flexibility in thinking by using card sorting

8. A test of non-verbal memory and constructional abilities

9. A test of motor sequencing

NEUROLOGICAL EXAMINATION

Theme: Eye signs encountered in clinical practice

Options for questions: 10–12

A   Argyll Robertson pupil
B   Holmes–Adie pupil
C   Hutchinson's pupil
D   Marcus Gunn pupil

E   Senile pupil
F   Horner's syndrome (unilateral constricted pupil)

For each of the following presentations, select the single most likely eye sign. Each option may be used once, more than once or not at all.

10. The pupils demonstrate sluggish light and accommodation reflexes.

11. The pupil on one side constricts and then dilates widely. The pupil on the other side goes through the same sequence.

12. When light is swung from eye to eye, dwelling for 2–3 seconds on each, the affected pupil eventually paradoxically dilates.

Theme: Diagnosis of uncommon psychiatric syndromes

Options for questions: 13–16

A   Angular gyrus syndrome
B   Anton's syndrome
C   Bálint's syndrome
D   Ganser's syndrome

E   Klüver–Bucy syndome
F   Korsakoff's syndrome
G   Ramsay Hunt syndrome

For each of the following cases, select the single most likely syndrome. Each option may be used once, more than once or not at all.

13. A 45-year-old man presented with a history of stroke. He was unable to direct voluntary eye movements at visual targets. He also had visual disorientation and visual attention deficit.

14. A 70-year-old woman presented with an inability to identify objects placed in her visual field. She denied that she was blind and made guesses for the questions related to objects in the visual field.

15. A 66-year-old man presented with a history of stroke. He was unable to name fingers. He could not correctly identify the right or left side of the body. He also had difficulty making simple calculations.

16. A 55-year-old man presented with a history of alcohol dependence. He was involved in a road traffic accident recently. He told stories about his past, some of which were not true. He filled memory gaps with fantastic stories. His implicit memory was intact.

ASSESSMENT

Theme: Assessment of alcohol-related sequelae

Options for questions: 17–19

A   Acquired immune deficiency syndrome
B   Comorbid opiate overdose
C   Delirium tremens
D   Intracranial bleed

E   Korsakoff's psychosis
F   Malingering
G   Wernicke's encephalopathy

For each of the following cases, select the single most likely alcohol-related sequela. Each option may be used once, more than once or not at all.

17. A 45-year-old man presented himself to the accident and emergency department (A&E). He was aggressive and smelt strongly of alcohol. He had a cut on his head and displayed fluctuating levels of consciousness. He was restless and agitated, and complained of seeing squirrels, insects and frightening faces around him.

18. A 61-year-old man presented to A&E. On examination, he was found to be ignoring the left side of his body.

19. A 31-year-old man presented to A&E. On examination, he had constricted pupils, bradycardia, and abscesses in both groins and the neck region.

AETIOLOGY

Theme: Suicide and mental disorder

Options for questions: 20–23

A	3%	F	45%
B	10%	G	55%
C	15%	H	65%
D	25%	I	70%
E	35%		

In Barraclough et al (1974), a historical study of 100 cases of suicide was investigated retrospectively by interviewing surviving relatives. The percentage of patients who had a mental health diagnosis before committing suicide was recorded. For each of the following disorders, select the single most likely percentage of patients. Each option may be used once, more than once or not at all.

20. Alcoholism

21. Anxiety disorder

22. Depressive disorder

23. No mental illness

DIAGNOSIS

Theme: Diagnosis of motor disorders

Options for questions: 24–26

A	Akathisia	E	Echopraxia
B	Catalepsy	F	Mannerism
C	Cataplexy	G	Stereotypes
D	Dystonia	H	Tardive dyskinesia

For each of the following cases, select the single most likely motor disorder. Each option may be used once, more than once or not at all.

24. A 55-year-old married woman with a long history of schizophrenia presented to the outpatient clinic for review. Her mental state has remained stable for 5 years on regular antipsychotic medication. However, over the past year her husband has noticed that she frequently makes faces and grimaces at him and other family members.

25. A 50-year-old happily married woman presents to A&E after a fall. She has a history of recurrent falls to the ground often after excitement or laughter. Physical examination reveals no apparent abnormalities.

26. A 30-year-old man with learning disabilities and schizophrenia lives in a care home. He spends a lot of time in a chair rocking back and forth when he is at home.

Theme: Differential diagnosis (or ICD-10) of common mental disorders

Options for questions 27–29

A Acute and transient psychotic disorder, unspecified
B Bipolar affective disorder, current episode of severe depression with psychotic symptoms
C Mental and behavioural disorder due to use of psychoactive drugs
D Moderate depressive episode
E Postpsychotic depression
F Prolonged depressive reaction
G Pseudodementia
H Schizoaffective disorder, depressive type
I Schizophrenia
J Severe depressive episode with psychotic symptoms

For each of the following cases, select the most likely diagnosis/diagnoses. Each option may be used once, more than once or not at all.

27. A 26-year-old man presented for the first time with a history of hearing voices calling his name over the last 4 weeks. He broke up with his partner 2 months earlier. His family had noticed that he had been withdrawn and socially isolated for 6 months. He used to smoke cannabis occasionally until 6 months ago and has tested negative for the drug (select TWO options).

28. A 49-year-old man presented for the first time complaining of low mood, difficulty in falling asleep, loss of appetite, poor concentration and impaired short-term memory for the past 3 months. He reported that he could hear his name being called out when he drifted off to sleep but not at other times. He also said that he had felt things going wrong since he left his wife 4 months ago (select TWO options).

29. A 72-year-old woman with a history of five admissions since she was 50 was readmitted to the hospital. She had not been eating or drinking for the past week. She was mute and uncooperative. Before the admission, she had been telling her family that she had no money or clothes, had committed a serious fraud and deserved to die (select ONE option).

CLASSIFICATION

Theme: Psychosomatic presentations in clinical practice

Options for questions: 30–32

A Adjustment disorder
B Hypochondriasis
C Illness behaviour
D Sick role
E Somatisation disorder
F Type A behaviour
G Type B behaviour

For each of the following cases, select the single most likely diagnosis. Each option may be used once, more than once or not at all.

30. A 52-year-old, previously healthy man had developed chest pains and dizziness. He went to his general practitioner who did some tests and advised him to follow a low-fat diet and undertake moderate exercise; was prescribed some tablets and given a sick note for 3 weeks. He was fully compliant with his treatment and was keen to return to work as soon as possible.

31. A 55-year-old man's colleagues felt that his heart problems were to be expected, considering his high ambition-driven behaviour and tendency to be abrupt with others.

32. A 53-year-old man developed chest pains and dizzy spells. All relevant investigations were normal. However, over the following few weeks, he started feeling anxious, depressed and unable to cope with life.

Theme: ICD-10 diagnosis of childhood and adolescence disorders

Options for questions: 33–37

A   Conduct disorder

B   Disorders of social functioning with onset specific to childhood and adolescence

C   Emotional disorders with onset specific to childhood

D   Hyperkinetic disorder

E   Mixed disorders of conduct and emotions

F   Oppositional defiant disorder

G   Other behavioural disorders and emotional disorders with onset usually occurring in childhood and adolescence

H   Pervasive development disorders

I   Specific development disorders of scholastic skills

J   Specific development disorders of mental function

K   Tic disorders

For each of the following diagnostic guidelines, select the single most likely disorder. Each option may be used once, more than once or not at all.

33. A 10-year-old boy presented with persistently negative, hostile, defiant, proactive and disruptive behaviour, which was outside the normal range.

34. A 34-year-old female doctor informed her medical student that normal or near-normal early development was followed by partial or complete loss of acquired hand skills and speech, together with deceleration in head growth.

35. A 23-year-old medical student discussed specific and significant impairment in the development of acquisition of skills in the absence of a history of a specific reading disorder. This was not due to low mental age, a visual acuity problem or inadequate schooling. The ability to spell orally and to write out words correctly was affected.

36. An 8-year-old boy presented with markedly defiant, disobedient and proactive behaviour with an absence of severe aggression.

37. A 12-year-old girl attended with her mother to discuss her problem with nail-biting.

NEUROTIC DISORDERS

Theme: Differential diagnosis of generalised anxiety disorders

Options for questions: 38–42

A	Body dysmorphophobia	E	Post-traumatic stress disorder
B	Hypochondriacal disorder	F	Somatisation disorder
C	Obsessive–compulsive disorder	G	Specific phobia
D	Panic disorder		

For each of the following cases, select the single most likely diagnosis. Each option may be used once, more than once or not at all.

38. A 32-year-old woman suffers from the disorder that is included in the subcategories of other anxiety disorders.

39. A 56-year-old woman experienced repetitive thoughts for 2 weeks, which were followed by ritualistic behaviours.

40. A 36-year-old woman presented with a history of 2 years of multiple symptoms. She had a preoccupation with complaints of physical symptoms.

41. A 47-year-old man presented with a preoccupation with serious physical disease for the last 6 months. He persistently refused to accept medical assurance.

42. A 19-year-old woman presented with a preoccupation with bodily disfigurement for the past year.

BASIC PSYCHOPHARMACOLOGY

Theme: Side effects of psychotropic drugs

Options for questions: 43–45

A	Akathisia	F	Hypothyroidism
B	Breathlessness	G	Insomnia
C	Coarse tremor	H	Nausea
D	Diabetes insipidus	I	Syndrome of inappropriate antidiuretic
E	Diarrhoea		hormone secretion

For each of the following cases, select the most likely side-effect(s) to be watched out for. Each option may be used once, more than once or not at all.

43. A 37-year-old man was commenced on lithium for bipolar affective disorder (select TWO options).

44. A 49-year-old woman presented with a history of first episode depression. She was prescribed citalopram. She was reviewed in the outpatient clinic 4 weeks later (select TWO options).

45. A 19-year-old man was admitted to the ward with his first acute psychotic episode. He was prescribed oral risperidone (select ONE option).

HUMAN PSYCHOLOGICAL DEVELOPMENT

Theme: Concepts associated with Jean Piaget

Options for questions: 46–48

A	Accommodation	F	Hypothetico-deductive reasoning
B	Animism	G	Laws of conservation
C	Assimilation	H	Object permanence
D	Circular reaction	I	Propositional thought
E	Egocentrism	J	Syncretism

For each of the following cases, select the single most likely concept from Piaget's theory. Each option may be used once, more than once or not at all.

46. A 2-year-old boy lost his ball under the covers and forgets about it, then moved on to play with another toy, behaving as if the first toy never existed.

47. A 13-year-old girl can cope with the discussion about 'what would happen if water ran uphill.'

48. A 4-year-old boy is able to consider the world only from his own viewpoint.

DESCRIPTION AND MEASUREMENT

Theme: Attributes of rating scales

Options for questions: 49–51

A	Concurrent validity	D	Inter-rater reliability
B	Content validity	E	Predictive validity
C	Criterion validity	F	Test-re-test validity

For each of the following descriptions, select the single most likely attribute of the scale being tested. Each option may be used once, more than once or not at all.

49. A group of clinicians and former patients was asked to give their opinion on whether they were being asked appropriate questions about the level of satisfaction of treatment received in an outpatient clinic.

50. An audit of patients who received treatment for depression was conducted to investigate whether their bas-line rating scale was related to their mental state.

51. A group of patients was asked to complete a personality rating scale 1 year apart.

DESCRIPTIVE PSYCHOPATHOLOGY

Theme: Sleep disorders

Options for questions: 52–54

A   Automatism
B   Bruxism
C   Night terrors
D   Nightmares

E   Nocturnal enuresis
F   Sleep apnoea
G   Somnambulism

For each of the following cases, select the single most likely sleep disorder. Each option may be used once, more than once or not at all.

52. A 50-year-old happily married man punched his wife badly while asleep but has no recollection of it the following morning.

53. A 12-year-old boy, while asleep, sat up suddenly in his bed terrified, but he had no recollection of doing this the following morning.

54. A 35-year-old man, on waking, believed that he had been beaten up by someone during the night, although there was no evidence to support this.

Theme: Disorders of perception

Options for questions: 55–57

A   Autoscopy
B   Completion illusion
C   Dysmegalopsia
D   Extracampine hallucination

E   Functional hallucination
F   Pareidolia
G   Reflex hallucination
H   Synaesthesia

For each of the following cases, select the single most likely perceptual disorder. Each option may be used once, more than once or not at all.

55. A 39-year-old man described seeing a black colour when he listens to the radio and a red colour when he watches television.

56. A 19-year-old man with schizophrenia describes being able to see a picture of angels when he looks at flowery wallpaper.

57. A 73-year-old man with psychotic depression described repeatedly hearing derogatory voices about him in a supermarket, a mile from the hospital where he was recently an inpatient.

DYNAMIC PSYCHOPATHOLOGY

Theme: Ego defence mechanisms

Options for questions: 58–60

A Denial
B Displacement
C Idealisation
D Identification

E Projective identification
F Rationalisation
G Reaction formation

For each of the following cases, select the single most likely defence mechanism. Each option may be used once, more than once or not at all.

58. A 39-year-old British man was attacked by a shark while swimming in the sea in South Africa. He lost both legs below the knee joint and required bilateral amputation. He talked animatedly about his holiday and did not answer when asked about recent events.

59. A 21-year-old man was recently detained under mental health legislation. Since then he has become very aggressive towards the domestic staff but pleasant to the doctors who detained him.

60. A 30-year-old man's father died unexpectedly a few weeks ago. He had had a hedonistic lifestyle previously but lived at home again. He now applied for a job at his father's company.

HISTORY OF PSYCHIATRY

Theme: Pioneers in psychological theories and concepts

Options for questions: 61–66

A Albert Bandura
B BF Skinner
C Clark L Hull
D David Premack
E Edward L Thorndike
F Harry Harlow

G Ivan Pavlov
H John B Watson
I Jean Piaget
J John Bowlby
K Mary Ainsworth

For each of the following concepts, select the single person most likely to be involved. Each option may be used once, more than once or not at all.

61. Magical thinking

62. Infant attachment and separation

63. Strange situation procedure

64. Operant conditioning

65. Conservation

66. Syllogistic reasoning

Answers: EMIs

1. A Advanced sleep phase syndrome

In advanced sleep phase syndrome, the patient complains of evening sleepiness, early sleep onset and early morning awakening. In contrast to depression, sleep is continuous, without awakenings, the patient feels refreshed and the total sleep time is normal for age. It is more prevalent in elderly people.

2. F Rhythmic movement disorder

Rhythmic movement disorder is characterised by stereotyped, repetitive movement involving large muscles, usually of the head and neck. It occurs typically immediately before sleep and is sustained into light sleep. This disorder is more common in young children and occurs more frequently in boys. Treatment is not necessary in most cases and it resolves in most children by the age of 18 months.

3. E Non-24-hour sleep–wake disorder

Patients with non-24-hour sleep–wake disorder will have an 'in-phase' period when they are free of symptoms every few weeks. This should alert the clinician to the possibility of this rare condition. There is a reported association with schizoid personality traits. Although its prevalence in blind people is unknown, one survey revealed a high incidence of a sleep–wake cyclical pattern in 40% of the respondents.

An irregular sleep–wake pattern, delayed sleep phase syndrome, shift-work sleep disorder and time zone change (jet lag) syndrome are dyssomnias–circadian rhythm sleep disorders.

4. A Closed questions

These are usually geared towards some factual response that has little room for debate. If there is over-reliance on this style of interviewing, it leads to failure to facilitate free expression.

5. C Normalising statement

Normalising is a technique for eliciting sensitive information; it is done by implying that it is understandable or by describing others who have had the experience.

6. E Polythematic questioning

Polythematic questioning or 'run on' refers to the process of asking the patient a number of questions simultaneously.

7. A Berg (1948)

The Wisconsin card sorting test was developed by DA Grant and EA Berg (1948). It is a test of basic abstract thinking and the ability to shift simple mental sets. The test requires participants to match ('sort') a set of 128 cards according to colour, shape or number. Intermittently the participant is corrected while using a sorting strategy, and at that point must recognise that he or she needs to shift the response set.

8. F Rey (1964)

The Rey–Osterrieth complex figure test involves showing a complex figure to the participant who is asked to copy it. The original and copy are then removed and the participant is asked to draw the figure again from memory at varying intervals to test–re-test reliability after a re-test interval was reported as 0.76 for immediate recall and 0.89 for delayed recall.

9. E Luria (1996)

Motor sequencing in battery consists of 269 items arranged in 14 scales which give information on motor, tactile, auditory and intellectual functioning, as well as receptive and expressive language abilities.

10. B Holmes–Adie pupil

This is also called myotonic pupil. It is usually a dilated pupil and is seen most commonly in young women. It is usually unilateral and often irregular. It is due to denervation of unknown cause in the coeliac ganglion. It is often associated with diminished or absent tendon reflexes.

11. D Hutchinson's pupil

It is a clinical sign in which the pupil on the side of an intracranial mass lesion is dilated and non-reactive to light because of the pressure on the occulomotor nerve of that side.

12. E Marcus Gunn pupil

This is a relative afferent pupillary defect indicating a decreased pupillary response to light in the affected eye. It is seen in optic neuritis and retrobulbar optic neuritis due to multiple sclerosis.

An Argyll Robertson pupil is small, irregular (3 mm or less) and fixed to light, but constricts on convergence. It is almost diagnostic of neurosyphillis. It is due to a lesion in the brain stem, in the neural tissue surrounding the sylvian aqueduct.

Horner's syndrome is characterised by unilateral papillary constriction with a slight relative ptosis and enophthalmos; it and is indicative of a lesion of the sympathetic pathway on the same side.

13. C Bálint's syndrome

This is characterised by a triad of symptoms of simultanagnosia, which is the inability to see the whole picture, optic ataxia and ocular apraxia. It is a type of cortical blindness in which a patient can see small visual details but fail to perceive the whole object, i.e. the ' patient cannot see the forest for the trees'. It is commonly seen with bilateral lesions, usually not involving the visual cortex.

14. B Anton's syndrome

This is also known as the Anton–Babinski syndrome and is due to lesions in the occipital lobe. It is characterised by occipital, cortical blindness, anosognosia and confabulation. Anton emphasised that a loss of neurological function may not be perceived by the person if the brain lesion occurs in a region known to be important for that function; the lesions are associated with bilateral cortical lesions that are 'almost symmetrical'.

15. A Angular gyrus syndrome

The Gerstmann–Sträussler–Scheinker syndrome is also known as the angular gyrus syndrome. It is characterised by right–left disorientation, finger agnosia, acalculia (difficulty with number reading, number writing or calculations), and agraphia of the central or linguistic type.

16. F Korsakoff's syndrome

Korsakoff's syndrome is due to chronic alcohol misuse, memory disturbance and confabulation.

Ganser's syndrome is characterised by approximate answers. It is usually seen in prisoners.

The Klüver–Bucy syndrome is due to bilateral temporal lobe injury. Its clinical features include hyperorality, hypersexuality, tameness and hypermetamorphosis, i.e. irresistible impulse to respond to every stimulus, and visual agnosia.

The Ramsay Hunt syndrome is due to a viral illness (varicella-zoster). Its clinical features include seventh nerve palsy, deafness and vertigo.

17. C Delirium tremens

This occurs in patients who are severely dependent on alcohol and have stopped or reduced their drinking. It is characterised by marked tremor of the limbs, body and tongue, restlessness, the clouding of consciousness, a loss of contact with reality, and illusions that progress to terrifying hallucinations, most commonly visual but possibly auditory and tactile.

18. D Intracranial bleed

Sustainance of a head injury while in a drunken state, which leads to an intracranial bleed, is likely.

19. B Comorbid opiate overdose

Such an overdose produces respiratory depression, constricted pupils, constipation and bradycardia.

20. E 15%

Fifteen per cent of people who end their own life have a diagnosis of alcoholism. An alcohol-dependent person has a continuing lifetime risk of suicide of about 7%. The risk of suicide is high in men, older age groups, people with a long history of drinking, and a previous history of depression and suicide attempts. The risk of suicide is high among people with physical complications, marital problems, work-related problems and difficulties with the law.

21. B 3%

About 3% of people who take their own life have a diagnosis of anxiety disorder. In these, the most striking features include the mental and physical symptoms of anxiety, generally in the absence of organic brain disease or another mental disorder.

22. K 70%

About 70% of patients who commit suicide have been treated for depression. It is found that about 6% of patients suffering from a mood disorder will take their own life. These patients are more likely to have a past history of self-harm. They have been noted to have experienced a sense of hopelessness and helplessness. These patients are often single, separated, or widowed, older men.

23. B 3%

In a historic retrospective study, Barraclough et al (1974) interviewed surviving relatives of 100 cases of suicide and found that 93% were diagnosed with mental illness. Of these, 80% were under doctors' follow-up, 80% were on psychotropic medication and over half had given a warning of suicidal thinking.

The findings were as follows: depressive disorder 70%, alcoholism 15%, anxiety disorder 3%, schizophrenia 3%, no mental disorder 7% and other diagnosis 2%.

Subsequent suicidal studies, e.g. Lonnqvist JK (2000) found a different result; 80–90% of the suicide cases had a DSM axis 1 diagnosis.

The findings were as follows:

Depressive disorder 32%, substance-related disorder 20%, personality disorder 10%, anxiety disorder 10%, schizophrenia 9%, no mental disorder 5%, bipolar 3% and organic disorder 1%.

24. H Tardive dyskinesia

This is characterised by repetitive purposeless movements usually of mouth, tongue and facial muscles; and possibly akathisia. It is more common among women, the elderly and patients with diffuse brain pathology. Clinically, it presents as chewing and sucking movements, grimacing and choreoathetoid movements.

25. C Cataplexy

This is sudden and transient loss of muscle tone precipitated by intense emotions such as anger, surprise, excitement and laughter. Cataplexy can present as weakness of the facial muscles, knees or more widespread weakness leading to falls lasting for few seconds to couple of minutes. The patient is fully conscious and aware of their surroundings. Cataplexy is usually seen in narcolepsy.

26. G Stereotypes

A stereotyped posture is abnormal and non-adaptive and maintained rigidly. Verbal stereotypes are words or phrases that are repeated.

27. I, J Schizophrenia; severe depressive episode with psychotic symptoms

Given the brief history, there are two diagnostic possibilities in this vignette.

28. D, F Moderate depressive episode; prolonged depressive reaction

Given the brief history, there are two diagnostic possibilities in this vignette.

29. J Severe depressive episode with psychotic symptoms

Given the brief history, the diagnosis is severe depressive episode with psychotic symptoms.

30. D Sick role

Society bestows a special role on people who are ill. Parsons called this the 'sick role' which is made up of two privileges and two roles: exemption from certain social responsibilities; the right to expect help and care from others; the obligation to seek and cooperate with treatment; and the expectation of a desire to recover.

31. F Type A behaviour

This is a complex of distinct traits such as aggressiveness, ambitiousness, competitiveness, impatience, cynicism, which are time pressured and achievement oriented. People with this behaviour type are prone to myocardial infarction and angina. It may be that hostility is associated with the risk of coronary heart disease. Their self-esteem often depends on constant achievement. Many physicians believe that modifying a type A behaviour pattern is an integral part of preventing future myocardial infarctions. Type B behaviour pattern is a cluster of behaviour including a relaxed attitude, indifference to time pressure and less forceful ambition, and was originally thought to be low risk for heart disease. It is characterised by inhibition of negative emotions, and avoiding contact with others. Type A personality may be at increased risk of cardiovascular morbidity and mortality, and cortisol may be a mediating factor for this increased risk.

32. A Adjustment disorder

This refers to a psychological reaction arising in relation to adapting to new circumstances. The patient is in a state of subjective distress and emotional disturbance, which usually interferes with social functioning and performance. This disorder arises during a period of adaptation to a significant life change or a stressful life event such as a bereavement or separation. An individual's predisposition or vulnerability plays an important role in the risk of the occurrence and shaping of symptoms of adjustment disorders. These disorders can manifest as depressed mood, anxiety, worry or a mixture of these, and a feeling of an inability to cope, plan ahead or manage daily chores.

33. A Conduct disorder

This is characterised by a repetitive and persistent pattern of dissocial, aggressive or defiant conduct. Such behaviour should amount to major violations of age-appropriate behaviour and social expectations. It should persist for at least 6 months. It can also be secondary to other mental disorders. Examples include excessive fighting or bullying, cruelty to other people or animals, firesetting, stealing, repeated lying, truancy or disobedience.

34. H Pervasive development disorder

Pervasive development disorder (Rett's syndrome) is found exclusively in girls. Its onset is usually between 7 and 24 months of age. An apparently normal early development is followed by partial or complete loss of speech, locomotor skills and use of hands, and a deceleration in head growth. Loss of purposive hand movements, hand-wringing stereotypies and hyperventilation are characteristic features. Truncal ataxia and apraxia start to develop by age 4. Choreoathetoid movements frequently follow. Initially social interests tend to be maintained. Severe learning disability almost invariably results.

35. I Specific development disorders of scholastic skills

In a specific spelling disorder, a person finds difficulty in spelling the words orally and also makes mistakes while writing. It is important to ascertain that person does not have a specific reading disorder, learning disability or problems with vision. The score on a standardised spelling test is at least 2 standard deviations below the expected level for that child. Interestingly scores on reading accuracy and comprehension and on arithmetic are within the normal range, i.e. +/– 2 standard deviation from the mean.

36. F Oppositional defiant disorder

When a conduct disorder is present in younger children, it comes under oppositional defiant disorder (ODD). Children with this diagnosis are defiant, do not obey their parents and have disruptive behaviour. They do not present with an extreme form of aggression or behavior that is considered dissocial. To diagnose ODD, the behaviour must be present for more than 6 months.

37. G Other behavioural and emotional disorders with onset usually occurring in childhood and adolescence

Nail-biting is an example of this category, which is a heterogeneous group of disorders sharing the characteristic of an onset in childhood, but otherwise differing in many respects. Some of the disorders present with well-defined syndromes, but others are no more than symptom complexes which must be included because of their frequency and association with psychosocial problems.

38. G Specific phobia

Specific phobias are also known as isolated phobias. They are an extreme fear of some specific object or situation. Some examples are fear of dogs or spiders. A specific phobia can present as a fear of some specific situations such as heights, seeing blood or an injury. It also presents with avoidance behaviour. Generalised anxiety disorder, panic disorder, and mixed anxiety and depression are part of a subcategory of other anxiety disorders. They differ from phobic anxiety disorders as the latter manifest in well-defined situations whereas the former are not restricted to any environmental situation.

39. C Obsessive–compulsive disorder

In the ICD-10, obsessive–compulsive disorder (OCD) comes under neurotic, stress-related disorders. OCD is characterised by obsessions and compulsions that are present for a period of 2 weeks. It can be in the form of thoughts or acts that are compulsive. Thoughts are repetitive, intrusive and persistent, and don't make any sense to the person. They are present with anxiety and are egodystonic. OCD can present with repetitive acts such as washing, cleaning or counting. These acts are performed to neutralise the thoughts or doubts and are not enjoyed by the person.

40. F Somatisation disorder

This comes under somatoform disorder in the ICD-10. People with somatisation disorder have many physical symptoms which are present over and over again and change frequently. The duration of symptoms should be present for at least 2 years. Patients usually contact many doctors and go through many investigations, which are usually negative. It can present in any part of body and affect a person's socio-occupational functioning.

41. B Hypochondriasis disorder

This disorder is characterised by a persistent preoccupation with the possibility of having one or more serious and progressive physical illnesses which do not respond to reassurance. The patient presents with persistent somatic symptoms or a preoccupation with physical appearance. Comorbid conditions such as anxiety and depression are often present.

42. A Body dysmorphophobia

This is regarded by the ICD-10 as a subtype of hypochondriasis whereas the DSM-IV classifies it as a separate somatoform diagnosis. The essential feature is that the person is concerned about a defect in his or her appearance for which there is inadequate objective evidence. The person tries to hide the presumed defect and seeks reassurance from others about it. Comorbid depression is common. The affected person often attends doctors, especially plastic surgeons, in order to seek the desired alteration of their appearance.

43. E, H Diarrhoea; nausea

Lithium is a highly toxic ion and has the lowest margin of safety of any class of psychotropic drugs. The prevalence of most side effects is lower with 'slow'- or 'sustained'-release formulation which is the one now most commonly used. The most frequently reported adverse effects are gastrointestinal. It is usually possible to distinguish between the major effects that occur therapeutically and those that indicate toxicity, but an overlap exists.

44. G, H Insomnia; nausea

Gastrointestinal upset with nausea is the commonest adverse effect (25–35%). Vomiting and diarrhoea also occur with greater frequency than with other antidepressants. These effects develop early in exposure and tend to ease as a steady state of plasma concentration is reached. Hence they are likely to be mediated by local (gastrointestinal) rather than central actions.

45. A Akathisia

Antipsychotics can be associated with the production of a wide range of adverse effects. Despite this, as a class they are remarkably safe and have wide therapeutic use. Akathisia may occur within hours of oral, and within 30 minutes of parental, administration of an antipsychotic drug. Predisposing factors depend on the potency, dose and rate of increment. The syndrome of inappropriate antidiuretic hormone secretion is often drug induced, particularly by drugs that impair renal excretion of water. It is characterised by hyponatraemia and hypo-osmolality of the serum and extracellular fluid, with continuous renal excretion of sodium. Carbamazepine, amitriptyline, fluoxetine, haloperidol and chlorpromazine can cause hyponatraemia.

46. H Object permanence

The sensorimotor stage of cognitive development is characterised by a lack of object permanence. In this stage, the world is known through action and sensory information. The ability to hold on to an image of an object, once it has been removed from view, develops progressively during this stage.

47. I Propositional thought

Stage 4 (the formal operational stage) is characterised by the ability to formulate hypotheses and systematically test them, to arrive at answers to problems posed at a purely verbal level. The arguments used in certain discussions can be evaluated in terms of the internal consistency of the statements used. This is an example of propositional thought. The logic of a statement is being evaluated without a checklist against a real-life situation.

48. E Egocentrism

This means that preoperational children are unable to consider the world from any viewpoint other than their own. Piaget described four stages through which individuals pass during cognitive development. These are shown in the **Table 1.1**.

Table 1.1 Piaget's stages of cognitive development

Stage	Approximate age range (in years)	Concepts that occur during this stage
Sensorimotor	0–2	Object permanence
Preoperational	2–7	Syncretic thought, transductive reasoning and animism
		Centration
		Egocentrism
Concrete operational	7–11	Conservation
Formal operational	11 and onwards	Manipulation of ideas and propositions based simply on verbal statements

49. B Content validity

Validity is a property of an instrument that refers to whether a test measures what it is supposed to measure. Content validity refers to the representativeness and relevance of the assessment instrument to the construct being measured.

50. E Predictive validity

This refers to the degree to which a test predicts some criterion that might be achieved in the future.

51. F Test–re-test validity

Test–re-test validity refers to whether or not the instrument measures the same after an interval.

52. A Automatism

In automatism, an action takes place in the absence of consciousness. That means that a person has no control over his or her behaviour. Usually, the person does not remember his or her behaviour. An automatism does not relate to the circumstances or the situation in which it is carried out. The behaviour is purposeful but lacks judgement.

53. C Night terrors

These occur in deep sleep early in the night and often in individuals who sleepwalk. The person experiences intense, shouts and breathes heavily. Usually there is complete amnesia of the experience on waking, unlike nightmares.

54. D Nightmares

These occur in the lighter stages of sleep and are a type of unpleasant dream. The transfixed sensation of the nightmare is an accurate representation of the sleep paralysis that occurs in that phase.

55. H Synaesthesia

This is the experience of a stimulus on one sensory modality producing a sensory experience in another. Reflex hallucinations are a morbid form of synaesthesia in which a sensory stimulus in one sensory modality produces a hallucination in another.

56. F Pareidolia

This consists of vivid illusions that occur without the patient making any effort. The illusions are the result of excessive fantasy thinking and a vivid visual imagery. They cannot be explained as the result of affect or mind set

57. D Extracampine hallucination

An extracampine hallucination is one outside the limits of the sensory field.

58. A Denial

This is a primitive defence mechanism. It is defined as the expressed refusal to acknowledge a threatening reality. It can operate only in the undeveloped, infantile psyche or in people whose ego is weak or disturbed. In other words, it means remaining unaware of difficult events or subjective truths that are too hard to accept by pushing them into the unconscious.

59. B Displacement

This is a neurotic defence mechanism. It involves transferring the emotional response from a person to someone else who in some way resembles the original person, who is not associated with as much conflict or risk or is less threatening.

60. C Idealisation

This is a primitive defence mechanism. It means ascribing a characteristic to another person or organisation, e.g. excellence, beauty, positive qualities, perfection, omnipotence, omniscience, unfailing empathy, unswerving love, unparalleled competence. A repetition of the infantile idealisation process occurs often in the treatment of people with personality disorders.

61. I Jean Piaget

Magical thinking means a belief that certain actions and outcomes are connected, although there is no rational basis for establishing a connection (e.g. if a cat crosses your path, it will bring bad luck to you). It is common in normal children and is the basis for most superstitious beliefs.

62. J John Bowlby

Attachment refers to the strong emotional bond that exists between a child and a caregiver. It develops through appropriate, sensitive, parental responses to the child's behavioural cues. It allows the child to develop understanding of his or her 'inner world' and how to understand the world around him or her. There are secure, insecure avoidant, insecure anxious, insecure ambivalent and disorganised types of attachments.

63. K Mary Ainsworth

According to Mary Ainsworth, the attachment system is just one among several other innate systems proposed as operating in infancy. It is the interplay between competing behavioural systems that led to the gold standard measure of attachment in infancy. Mary Ainworth's strange situation procedure (SSP) pits the attachment system against the fear and exploration system, in a structured, unfamiliar situation composed of increased levels of stress. Observations are focused primarily on proximity-seeking and contact-maintaining behaviours during reunions with the caregiver. The SSP initially suggested three types of infant behaviour: insecure-avoidant, secure, and insecure-resistant.

64. B BF Skinner

In operant conditioning, it has been suggested that the organism affects the world and vice versa. The organism is a part of the process and has some controlling effect on how that process takes place. The behaviour occurs without any observable external stimulus. It is the organism's actions that drives learning rather than another's actions. The organism's response appears spontaneous and independent of any known stimulus. The underlying premise of operant conditioning is that reinforced behaviours are likely to continue and those that are not will become extinct or cease to occur.

65. I Jean Piaget

Children master the concept of conservation when they realise that the quantity or amount of a substance or group of objects remains unchanged when nothing has been added or substracted.

66. I Jean Piaget

In the preoperational stage, there are two types of magical thinking: phenomenalistic causality and animistic thinking.

- Phenomenalistic: events are thought to occur close to each other.
- Anismistic: there is a tendency to endow physical events and objects with life-like psychological attributes.
- Symbolisation: infants use mental symbols to use words – observed at 18 months.
- Syllogistic reasoning: logical conclusion is formed from two premises, e.g. all horses are mammals and all mammals are warm-blooded. Therefore, all horses are warm-blooded.
- Contact comfort: during this stage the monkey infant depends on its mother for nourishment but also for warmth and comfort.

Chapter 2

Test questions: 2

Questions: EMIs

HISTORY AND MENTAL STATE EXAMINATION

Theme: Interview techniques

Options for questions: 1–5

A	Clarification	G	Open question
B	Closed question	H	Polythematic question
C	Confrontation	I	Recapitulation
D	Empathy	J	Reflection
E	Facilitation	K	Summation
F	Interpretation	L	Sympathy

For each of the following questions, select the single most likely psychiatric interview technique. Each option may be used once, more than once or not at all.

1. Do you hear voices or noises?

2. You seem very irritable when you talk about it.

3. What brings you to the hospital today?

4. Yes, and then? Go on 'tell me more about it'.

5. Do you hear voices throughout the day and what do these voices say?

COGNITIVE ASSESSMENT

Theme: Disorders of speech

Options for questions: 6–9

A	Broca's aphasia	E	Pure word blindness
B	Conduction aphasia	F	Transcortical motor aphasia
C	Global aphasia	G	Transcortical sensory aphasia
D	Nominal aphasia	H	Wernicke's aphasia

For each of the following cases, select the single most likely speech disorder. Each option may be used once, more than once or not at all.

6. A 40-year-old man presented with non-fluent aphasia

7. A 35-year-old man with the diagnosis of schizophrenia presented with jargon aphasia.

8. A 49-year-old man presented with difficulty in speech; his fluency and comprehension were intact but his ability with repetition and naming was lost.

9. A 55-year-old woman presented with speech that had intact fluency and repetition, but her ability with comprehension and naming was lost.

NEUROLOGICAL EXAMINATION

Theme: Disorders of speech

Options for questions: 10–13

A	Aphonia	F	Paragrammatism
B	Echolalia	G	Parapraxis
C	Flight of ideas	H	Stilted speech
D	Logoclonia	I	*Vorbeireden*
E	Neologism		

For each of the following cases, select the single most likely speech disorder. Each option may be used once, more than once or not at all.

10. A 45-year-old man was involved in a road traffic accident a few days ago. Since then, he was suddenly unable to speak clearly although he started speaking in a whisper that was difficult to hear. When asked to speak louder, he appeared to make great efforts but was still barely audible.

11. When a 35-year-old man was asked 'What is the colour of the sky?', he replied 'green'. When he was asked 'How many legs does a horse have?', he replied 'five'.

12. A 47-year-old male company director was giving a presentation at a conference. In his introductory speech he remarked, 'Murder of these two companies is the best way to ensure survival in difficult times.'

13. A 10-year-old boy had his own words for things and expected others to know what he meant when he spoke.

ASSESSMENT

Theme: Assessment of motor symptoms/signs in psychotic patients

Options for questions: 14–16

A   Ambidextrous
B   Ambitendency
C   Automatic obedience
D   Catalepsy
E   Echopraxia
F   *Mitgehen*
G   Psychological pillow
H   Stereotype

For each of the following cases, select the single most likely psychopathology. Each option may be used once, more than once or not at all.

14. A 35-year-old man had had schizophrenia for many years. When his psychiatrist tried to greet him by shaking his hand, he initially put out his arm to shake hands, then withdrew it, and then extended it. He repeated this gesture at least 10 times in rapid succession before finally resting without reaching the psychiatrist's hand.

15. A 30-year-old single woman had schizophrenia and took her antipsychotic drug regularly. She attended the outpatient clinic for her 6-monthly reviews. When the psychiatrist touched the back of her left forearm with his forefinger, her arm moved up. On continued touching, her left upper arm stayed at shoulder level while the arm flexed at the elbow.

16. A 55-year-old single man had schizophrenia for several years. His mental state had remained stable on antipsychotic drugs. When his psychiatrist asked him to raise his right arm, he raised both arms and stood up with both arms raised. Every time he was asked to raise his right arm, he repeated this gesture.

AETIOLOGY

Theme: Suicide risk factors

Options for questions: 17–19

A   Bereavement
B   Childhood deprivation
C   Life skills
D   Onset of physical disease
E   Relationship conflict
F   Response to treatment

For each of the following factors below, select the single most likely suicide risk factor. Each option may be used once, more than once or not at all.

17. Dynamic factor

18. Stable factor

19. Static factor

DIAGNOSIS

Theme: ICD-10 diagnosis of common mental disorders

Options for questions: 20–22

A	Adjustment disorder	E	Generalised anxiety disorder
B	Bipolar affective disorder	F	Hypochondriasis
C	Emotionally unstable personality disorder (borderline type)	G	Post-traumatic stress disorder
		H	Somatisation disorder
D	Emotionally unstable personality disorder (impulsive type)		

For each of the following cases, select the single most likely diagnosis. Each option may be used once, more than once or not at all.

20. A 48-year-old married man was involved in a road traffic accident 3 weeks ago. He complained of depressed mood, panic attacks, insomnia, and a feeling of being unable to cope with his work and home situation.

21. A 44-year-old woman has visited her general practitioner on numerous occasions over the past 2 years. She had been complaining of a variety of physical symptoms, e.g. bloating, diarrhoea, aches and pains in her abdomen, chest, head and joints, and fatigue, tingling and numbness of her hands. All investigations had proved negative and she felt reassured.

22. A 23-year-old male medical student had been concerned that the sensation of his heart beat had altered. He had been thoroughly investigated by his general practitioner. He had visited two cardiologists but was convinced that something had been missed. He was seeking another specialist opinion.

Theme: ICD-10 diagnosis of somatoform and dissociative disorders

Options for questions: 23–25

A	Body dysmorphic disorder	F	Multiple personality disorder
B	Conversion disorder	G	Persistent somatoform pain disorder
C	Factitious disorder	H	Somatisation disorder
D	Hypochondriasis	I	Undifferentiated somatoform disorder
E	Malingering		

For each of the following cases, select the single most likely diagnosis. Each option may be used once, more than once or not at all.

23. A 45-year-old woman developed left-sided lower and right-sided upper limb weakness following the death of her mother a few weeks ago. Neurological assessment revealed no abnormalities.

24. A 53-year-old man repeatedly presented to his family doctor with chest pain, shortness of breath and paraesthesia in his left arm following the death of his father from myocardial infarction. He was convinced that he had 'heart disease' in spite of negative investigations and repeated reassurances from his doctor.

25. A 47-year-old married woman had a 10-year history of multiple and frequent symptoms of abdominal pain, bloated feeling, chest pains, dysmenorrhoea, copious vaginal discharge and fatigue. Multiple physical examinations and investigations had proved negative.

Theme: Diagnosis of personality disorders

Options for questions: 26–29

A   Anankastic personality disorder
B   Anxious personality disorder
C   Dissocial personality disorder
D   Emotionally unstable personality disorder
     (borderline type)
E   Emotionally unstable personality disorder
     (impulsive type)

F   Histrionic personality disorder
G   Paranoid personality disorder
H   Narcissistic personality disorder
I   Schizoid personality disorder
J   Schizotypal personality disorder

For each of the following cases, select the single most likely diagnosis. Each option may be used once, more than once or not at all.

26. A 29-year-old woman presented with shallow and labile affect; she sought excitement and activities where she was centre of attention and was inappropriately seductive in her behaviour.

27. A 27-year-old man presented with excessive feelings of doubts, perfectionism, checking and preoccupation with details.

28. A 30-year-old house wife presented with persistent feelings of tension, apprehension, a feeling of being inferior to others and avoidance of social activities.

29. A 25-year-old woman with a tendency to act unexpectedly without caring about the consequences presented with frequent outbusts of anger and violence. She was quarrelsome and got upset easily.

BASIC PSYCHOPHARMACOLOGY

Theme: Mechanism of side effects of antipsychotic drugs

Options for questions: 30–32

A   Akathisia
B   Blurred vision
C   Constipation
D   Delayed ejaculation
E   Hyperprolactinaemia

F   Hypothermia
G   Postural hypotension
H   Prolonged QT interval
I   Urinary retention
J   Weight gain

For each of the following receptor blockades, select the most likely side effect as instructed. Each option may be used once, more than once or not at all.

30. D_2-receptor-like blockade (select THREE options).

31. Acetylcholine blockade (select THREE options).

32. Noradrenergic α_1-receptor blockade (select TWO options).

BASIC PSYCHOLOGICAL PROCESSES

Theme: Emotions

Options for questions: 33–36

A	Cannon and Bard	E	James-Lange
B	Darwin	F	Pavlov
C	Ekman	G	Schachler and Singer
D	Fish	H	Skinner

For each of the following descriptions, select the single person most likely to be involved. Each option may be used once, more than once or not at all.

33. The expression of emotion in man: stated that particular emotional responses, e.g. facial expressions, tend to accompany the emotions in humans of all races and cultures, even those who are born blind.

34. The subjective emotion is quite independent of psychological changes. The thalamus processes the emotion-producing stimulus and sends the information to the cortex, where emotion is consciously experienced, and to the hypothalamus which sets in motion the autonomic psychological changes.

35. Cognitive labelling of emotions.

36. Peripheralist theory of emotion.

HUMAN PSYCHOLOGICAL DEVELOPMENT

Theme: Piaget's stages of cognitive development

Options for questions: 37–40

A	Animism	G	Logical thought
B	Circular reaction	H	Object permanence
C	Conservation	I	Propositional thought
D	Egocentrism	J	Syncretism
E	Hypothetico-deductive reasoning	K	Transductive reasoning
F	Lack of conservation		

For each of the following stages of Piaget's cognitive development, select the two most likely concepts. Each option may be used once, more than once or not at all.

37. Concrete operational stage

38. Formal operational stage

39. Preoperational stage

40. Sensorimotor stage

SOCIAL PSYCHOLOGY

Theme: Neuropsychological tests

Options for questions: 41–44

A   Test of face processing
B   Test of language function
C   Test of reading ability
D   Test of working memory

E   Test of writing ability
F   Tests for unilateral neglect
G   Test of visual object agnosias

For each of the following neuropsychological tests, select the single most likely use of the test. Each option may be used once, more than once or not at all.

41. Letter or star cancellation tests

42. Peabody picture vocabulary test

43. Single-letter identification

44. Spontaneous writing of sentences

DESCRIPTION AND MEASUREMENT

Theme: Assessment of personality

Options for questions: 45–48

A   16 Personality factor questionnaire
B   Draw-a-person test
C   Eysenck personality questionnaire
D   Minnesota multiphasic personality inventory

E   Personality diagnostic questionnaire IV
F   Rorschach's test
G   Sentence completion test
H   Thematic apperception test

For each of the following descriptions, select the single most likely test that describes it best. Each option may be used once, more than once or not at all.

45. This instrument was developed through factor analysis. It measures dimensions of introversion, extroversion, psychoticism and social desirability.

46. This instrument was developed empirically with the original intent to create a measure of psychopathology. It provides scores on 10 clinical domains.

47. This instrument consists of 10 symmetrical inkblots and participants are asked to describe them.

48. This instrument consists of 20 cards presenting vague pictures on black and white blank cards. The participants are asked to create a story to fit each picture and explain what led up to the event in the picture.

DESCRIPTIVE PSYCHOPATHOLOGY

Theme: Disorders of perception

Options for questions: 49–51

A   Autoscopic hallucination
B   Delusional perception
C   *Écho de la pensée*
D   Elementary hallucination

E   Extracampine hallucination
F   *Gedankenlautwerden*
G   Hypnagogic hallucination
H   Hypnopompic hallucination

For each of the following cases, select the single most likely psychopathology. Each option may be used once, more than once or not at all.

49. A 19-year-old man complained that his friends anticipated his thoughts and spoke them out loud just before he could think of them.

50. A 45-year-old woman complained of being very frightened as she could hear a bell tolling wherever she was.

51. A 31-year-old woman believed that she had been bewitched because she could see herself in front of where she was standing.

Theme: Disorders of perception

Options for questions: 52–54

A   Affect illusion
B   Autoscopic hallucination
C   Eidetic imagery
D   Elementary hallucination
E   Extracampine hallucination

F   Haptic hallucination
G   Hyperschemazia
H   Paraschemazia
I   Pareidolia

For each of the following cases, select the single most likely perceptual disorder. Each option may be used once, more than once or not at all.

52. A 36-year-old woman described being able to see an intense, detailed picture even when there was nothing there. She could also make it go away.

53. A 17-year-old girl became convinced that she had a twin for a few minutes at a time. She often saw herself sitting just in front of where she was.

54. A 78-year-old woman described seeing several noisy people sitting behind her. However, when she turned around they would disappear.

BASIC ETHICS AND PHILOSOPHY OF PSYCHIATRY

Theme: Ethical principles in clinical practice

Options for questions: 55–58

A   Autonomy
B   Beneficence
C   Empiricism
D   Justice

E   Non-maleficence
F   Paternalism
G   Therapeutic privilege
H   Utilitarianism

For each of the following cases, select the single most likely ethical principle that describes it best. Each option may be used once, more than once or not at all.

55. The psychiatrist informed a 55-year-old man with Alzheimer's disease about his diagnosis, treatment and prognosis to enable him to make decisions about the future.

56. The psychiatrist informed a 78-year-old woman with Alzheimer's disease that the best thing to do to enable her to have a good quality of life was to go into a care home. In order not to make it too complex for her, the psychiatrist did not explain her other alternatives.

57. The psychiatrist decided not to tell a 72-year-old man with Alzheimer's disease about his diagnosis and prognosis despite the request to do so. The psychiatrist had judged that the patient was too emotionally unstable to cope with the consequences of his illness and that he might kill himself.

58. The psychiatrist who was treating a 64-year-old man with Alzheimer's dementia believed that prescribing antipsychotic medication to inpatients with behaviour problems was part of the requirement to do good to the patient.

Answers: EMIs

1. B Closed question

This is one of the directive techniques which includes when, how and what questions. Closed questioning expects a limited range of replies. In general, start the interview with open questions and proceed with more focused and closed questions to clarify the factual points.

2. F Interpretation

This means interpreting the situation, non-verbal and verbal communication with the patient and explaining it to him or her.

3. G Open question

Open-ended questions are used to initiate the interview and allow free narration. They usually start with 'Describe', 'Tell me', etc. They reflect an area for further exploration by the psychiatrist.

4. E Facilitation

This helps the patients to continue the conversation using verbal or non-verbal gestures to express interest. 'Yes', 'go-on', 'proceed', 'and then', 'uh-huh' are some of the facilitation techniques.

5. H Polythematic question

Reflections are repetitions of the patient's statements to let the patient know that the psychiatrist is taking an interest. Polythematic questioning, compound questioning or run-on questioning is an obstructive technique with two or more questions in a single statement confusing the patient.

6. A Broca's aphasia

Aphasia is a problem of language reception, production and processing. Most of the time aphasia is organic. Fluency depends on intact Broca's area and its forward connections. A defect in naming the objects is called anomia and it accompanies any aphasia to varying degrees. In Broca's motor aphasia, fluency, repetition and naming are lost but comprehension is intact.

7. H Wernicke's aphasia

Comprehension depends on intact Wernicke's area and it further connections with the association cortex and sensory input. In Wernicke's aphasia, fluency is intact but repetition, comprehension and naming are lost. Comprehension is lost for both spoken and written language. Language is fluent but highly paraphasic; sometimes neologisms and circumlocution are also seen, so it is also called jargon aphasia.

8. B Conduction aphasia

Sound is received by the ears and transmitted to Wernicke's area and auditory association cortex, which is responsible for processing the language component.

9. G Transcortical sensory aphasia

Repetition requires no higher level of functioning. Repetition can take place if Broca's area, Wernicke's area and arcuate fasciculus are intact. Therefore, in conduction aphasia, repetition and naming are lost but fluency and comprehension are intact.

In transcortical sensory aphasia, comprehension and naming are lost but fluency and repetition are intact.

10. A Aphonia

This is a common speech disorder. It can be complete (mutism) or incomplete when, within sounds produced there are usually no recognisable words at all. 'Mutism' is a condition in which the person does not speak or make attempt at spoken communication despite the preservation of an adequate level of consciousness.

11. I *Vorbeireden*

This is talking past the point, that is, the person understands what has been asked but has responded by talking about an associated topic. It occurs in dissociative/conversion disorder, i.e. Ganser's syndrome, and schizophrenia especially among adolescents and in catatonic states.

12. G Parapraxis

Freud applied the term 'parapraxis' to symptomatic acts such as slips of the tongue or mislaying of objects.

13. E Neologism

This may be new words that are constructed by the patient or ordinary words that are used in a new way. It is a term that is usually applied to new word formations produced by patients with schizophrenia.

14. B Ambitendency

This can be regarded as a mild variety of negativism or the result of obstruction. The patient makes a series of tentative movements that do not reach the intended goal when he or she is expected to carry out a voluntary action.

15. F *Mitgehen*

This can be regarded as an extreme form of cooperation because the patient moves his or her body in the direction of the slightest pressure by the examiner. When examining for *mitgehen* and cooperation, the patient must understand that he or she is expected to resist the examiner's efforts to move him or her.

16. C Automatic obedience

In this case, the patient carries out every instruction regardless of the consequence. Some psychiatrists have used the term 'command automatism' as a synonym for automatic obedience, waxy flexibility, echolalia and echopraxia.

17. E Relationship conflict

The dynamic factors are substance abuse, anxiety symptoms, relationship conflicts, cognitions and compliance with treatment.

18. C Life skills

The stable factors are age, enduring mental illness, personality, marital/parenting status and life skills.

19. B Childhood deprivation

Bouch and Marshall suggested that the static factors in suicide are gender, family background, history of overdose and childhood deprivation.

20. A Adjustment disorder

This is state of subjective distress and emotional disturbance, which usually interferes with social functioning and performance. It arises in a period of adaptation to a significant life change or a stressful life event.

21. H Somatisation disorder

The main features of somatisation disorder are multiple, recurrent and frequently changing physical symptoms of at least 2 years' duration. Most patients have a long and complicated history of contact with both primary and secondary medical care services. Its course is chronic and fluctuating.

22. F Hypochondriasis

The essential feature of hypochondriasis is a persistent preoccupation with the possibility of having one or more serious and progressive physical disorders. Patients manifest persistent somatic complaints or a persistent preoccupation with their physical appearance.

23. B Conversion disorder

The diagnosis of a conversion disorder should be made with great caution in the presence of physical disorders of the system, or in a previously well-adjusted individual with normal family and social relationships. The symptoms can often be seen to represent the patient's concept of physical disorders which may be at variance with physiological or anatomical principles.

24. A Body dysmorphic disorder

This is the DSM term for a subgroup of the broader, but ill-defined, clinical syndrome of dysmorphophobia. The typical patient with this disorder is convinced that some part of his or her body is too large, too small or misshapen. To other people, this is normal or the abnormality is trivial.

25. H Somatisation disorder

The main features of somatisation disorder are multiple, recurrent and frequently changing physical symptoms of at least 2 years' duration. Most patients have a long and complicated history of contact with both primary and secondary medical care services. Its course is chronic and fluctuating.

26. F Histrionic personality disorder

Histrionic personality disorder is characterised by shallow and labile affect, self-dramatisation, exaggerated expression of emotions, suggestibility, continual seeking for excitement, inappropriately seductive behaviour and overconcern about physical attractiveness.

27. A Anankastic personality disorder

Anankastic personality disorder is characterised by feelings of doubts, perfectionism, and preoccupation with the details, excessive conscientiousness, rigidity and stubbornness.

28. B Anxious personality disorder

Anxious personality disorder is characterised by persistent feelings of tension, the apprehension belief that they are inferior to others, unwillingness to involve with people, and restrictions in lifestyle because of the need for physical security.

29. E Emotionally unstable personality disorder (impulsive type)

Personality disorders are severe disturbances in one's personality and behavioural tendencies, which have not directly resulted from disease or damage to the brain. They are associated with significant distress at the personal and social levels. They usually manifest in childhood and continue throughout adolescence.

Emotionally unstable personality disorder is characterised by the tendency to act impulsively without considering the consequences. Mood is generally unpredictable. There is a tendency for emotional outbursts. It can be of the impulsive or borderline type. The impulsive type is characterised by a marked tendency to act unexpectedly, and to have quarrelsome behaviour and outbusts of anger and violence. Patients with this disorder have difficulty maintaining any course of action and an unpredictable mood. The borderline type is characterised by uncertainty or disturbance in self-image, a tendency to get into intense and unstable relationships, excessive efforts made to avoid abandonment, recurrent threats or acts of self-harm, and chronic feelings of emptiness.

30. A, E, J Akathisia; hyperprolactinaemia; weight gain

Akathisia is a compulsive motor restlessness, especially of the legs, usually accompanied by an unpleasant sense of mental agitation. It is a common reason for non-compliance with medication. It may also be linked to aggression, suicidal urges and behavioural disturbance. Some patients may show restless, non-goal-directed behaviour without feeling particularly agitated subjectively. This is best described as tardive akathisia.

Hyperprolactinaemia results from blockade of the tuberoinfundibular dopamine D_2-receptors. Rises in prolactin can be detected within a few hours of exposure, reaching a plateau within 4–7 days and staying elevated for the duration of exposure. Weight gain can be a major problem with all antipsychotics. The mechanism is unknown and multiple factors may be involved.

31. B, C, I Blurred vision; constipation; urinary retention

Dry mouth, constipation, blurred vision, urinary retention and sexual dysfunction are not uncommon complaints from patients taking antipsychotics. Some of the side effects are likely to have more complex origins than 'single transmitter' pharmacology. They may be at least partially mediated by antiadrenergic, as well as anticholinergic, mechanisms.

32. D, G Delayed ejaculation; postural hypotension

Antiautonomic actions of antipsychotics result in an increase in resting heart rate, usually of the order of 10 beats/min or less and not clinically significant. The antiadrenergic effects also produce a significant fall in blood pressure, which is mainly postural. This is a potentially serious problem that can precipitate myocardial ischaemia/infarction or a cerebrovascular accident.

33. B Darwin

Charles Darwin argued that certain complex actions are inherited and the role of instincts, through the process of natural selection, became influential in the developing discipline of psychology. Certain kinds of sensory experiences were innately rewarding and other activities gave inherent pleasure and satisfaction.

34. A Cannon and Bard

The centralist theory proposed by Cannon and Bard argued that physiology is casual. Significant stimuli activate the thalamus, which in turn generates both subjective responses and physiological signs of stress.

To summarise:

Emotional event → central brain system (thalamus)
                 → autonomic arousal
                 → emotion

35. G Schachler and Singer

According to the cognitive labelling theory proposed by Schachler and Singer, people label emotions using their perceptions of their own somatic activity. This is a cognitive process that is affected by the people's beliefs about the situation. If people believe that they have a reason to be angry, they will experience bodily symptoms such as anger and so forth.

36. E James-Lang

According to the peripheral list theory of emotion proposed by James-Lange, emotion is informed or constructed from instinctive peripheral physiological responses. Events provoke reflex bodily responses and emotions from the perception of those changes.

To summarise:

emotional event → preorganised mechanism
                 → peripheral bodily changes
                 → emotion

37. C, G Conservation; logical thought

Piaget described four stages through which individuals pass during cognitive development. These are shown in Table 2.1.

38. E, I Hypothetico-deductive reasoning; propositional thought

Piaget described four stages through which individuals pass during cognitive development. These are shown in Table 2.1.

39. A, D Animism; egocentrism

Piaget described four stages through which individuals pass during cognitive development. These are shown in Table 2.1.

40. B, H Circular reaction; object permanence

Piaget described four stages through which individuals pass during cognitive development. These are shown in Table 2.1.

Table 2.1 Piaget's stages of cognitive development		
Stage	**Approximate age range (in years)**	**Concepts that occur during this stage**
Sensorimotor	0–2	Object permanence
Preoperational	2–7	Syncretic thought, transductive reasoning and animism
		Centration
		Egocentrism
Concrete operational	7–11	Conservation
Formal operational	11 and onwards	Manipulates ideas and propositions simply on verbal statements

41. F Tests for unilateral neglect

Face processing is impaired in prosopagnosia. It is tested using photographs of faces or asking patients to describe emotions in pictures of different faces. Copying a drawing is usually used to detect visual object agnosia.

42. B Test of language function

Language functions have a wide range. One of the language function tests is the Peabody picture identification test.

43. C Test of reading ability

This test includes the national adult reading test (NART), reading a sentence and single letter identification. The NART has been the most widely used to estimate premorbid ability. It is a single-word, oral reading test consisting of 50 items. All the words are irregular, i.e. they violate grapheme–phoneme correspondence rules. As the words are irregular, intelligent guessing should not provide the correct pronunciation.

44. E Test of writing ability

This test uses spontaneous writing. Tests for unilateral neglect include clock drawing as well as the letter or star cancellation test. Working memory is tested using the digit-span test.

45. C Eysenck's personality questionnaire

This was devised by Hans Eysenckin 1975. He suggested that, to understand personality traits, we need to consider personality dimensions or dimensional traits which may vary from person to person. Each dimension is associated with personality traits that determine habitual responses. Extraversion–introversion refers to the degree to which a person's orientation is turned inward towards the self or outward towards the external world. Neuroticism–stability refers to people's emotionality. Psychoticism refers to aggression, coldness, eccentricity, impulsiveness, and antisocial and unempathatic behaviour.

46. D Minnesota multiphasic personality inventory

This provides scores on 10 clinical domains: hypochondrias, depression, hysteria, psychopathic deviate, masculinity/feminity, paranoia, psychasthenia, schizophrenia, hypomania and social introversion. The clinician can learn much more by looking at profiles and patterns than from looking at a single peak.

47. F Rorschach's test

This is a projective test of personality assessment which makes use of instructed stimuli. It consists of 10 symmetrical inkblocks and the patients have to describe them. It is thought that, when confronted with a vague stimulus, patients will introduce (project) some personality characteristics into the stimulus. This will be revealed not only in the way in which the ambiguity is perceived but also in the contents of their responses.

48. H Thematic apperception test

In this test, 20 stimulus cards depicting number scenes of varying ambiguity are used. In terms of the blank card, patients are asked to imagine a picture on the card, describe it and tell a story about it. The content of the stories is then analysed according to Murray's list of needs.

49. F *Gedankenlautwerden*

This is also known as thought echo or *écho de la pensée* and is an auditory hallucination in which the contents are the individual's current thoughts. The patient describes hearing thoughts spoken just before or at the same time as they are occurring. *Écho de la pensée* is the phenomenon of hearing them spoken after the thoughts have occurred. Patients may complain that their thoughts are no longer private but accessible to others.

50. D Elementary hallucination

This refers to experiences such as bangs, whistles and flashes of light. Complex hallucinations refer to experiences such as hearing voices or music, or seeing faces and scenes.

51. A Autoscopic hallucination

This is the experience of seeing one's own body projected into external space, usually in front of oneself for short periods. Healthy people in situations of sensory deprivation report the experience occasionally, when it is called an out-of-body or a near-death experience.

52. C Eidetic imagery

This represents visual memories of almost hallucinatory vividness. It is the awareness of a percept that has been generated within the mind. Imagery can be called up and terminated, by an effort of will. Eidetic imagery has 'photographic' quality akin to a percept, although in other ways it differs from a percept.

53. B Autoscopic hallucination

This is the experience of seeing one's own body projected into external space, usually in front of oneself for short periods. An extracampine hallucination is a hallucination that is outside the limits of the sensory field.

54. I Pareidolia

This involves vivid illusions, which occur without the patient making any effort. They are the result of excessive fantasy thinking and a vivid visual imagery. They cannot be explained as the result of affect or mindset.

55. A Autonomy

Respect for a patient's autonomy always heads the various short lists of prime prima facie ethical principles, reflecting the primary goal of the contractarian model. Accordingly, patients should be treated as autonomous agents who make their own decisions about their lives.

56. F Paternalism

This is a distortion of fatherly or parental behaviour, in which some moral rule relative to the actions of one person towards another is violated without the consent of the other person.

57. G Therapeutic privilege

Psychiatrists sometimes have to weigh up the pros and cons of disclosing facts to their patients. They then, on balance of probabilities, can decide to withhold information from their patients.

58. B Beneficence

The principle of beneficence relates to the requirement to do well or promote well-being. Non-maleficence relates to the requirement to do no harm. Hence, for almost all management plans and treatments, doctors have to make decisions based on a balance of benefits and harm. Hence, beneficence and non-maleficence are inseparable. However, depending on which principles doctors believe predominantly, it can lead to differing views and practice.

Chapter 3

Test questions: 3

Questions: EMIs

HISTORY AND MENTAL STATE EXAMINATION

Theme: Supportive and obstructive interventions during a psychiatric interview

Options for questions: 1–5

A	Acknowledging emotions	F	Non-verbal obstructive
B	Compound question	G	Non-verbal supportive
C	Dismissal	H	Premature advice
D	Encouragement	I	Reassurance
E	Judgemental	J	Trapping the patient in his or her own words

For each of the following scenarios, select the single most likely interview style. Each option may be used once, more than once or not at all.

1. A doctor said to a patient 'Even after many years, thinking about your dead father brings tears to your eyes'.

2. A doctor asked a patient, 'Do you feel depressed and do you have suicidal thoughts and ideas?'.

3. A 32-year-old man said to the doctor 'Over the last few months, I had trouble with sex' and the doctor replied with 'That happens from time to time'.

4. A 23-year-old woman said to her doctor 'I was not good at expressing my feelings' and the doctor replied 'I think you described things well and now I am able to better understand what you were going through'.

5. A 40-year-old woman informed her doctor 'I smoked cannabis sometimes' and the doctor replied 'Did you know that smoking cannabis can cause psychosis?'.

COGNITIVE ASSESSMENT

Theme: Cognitive examination

Options for questions: 6–10

A   Six-item recall
B   Ten-item recall
C   Attention and concentration
D   Clock-drawing test
E   Cognitive estimates
F   Frontal lobe
G   Motor fluency
H   Occipital lobe
I   Parietal lobe
J   Temporal lobe
K   Verbal fluency

For each of the following descriptions, select the single most likely option. Each option may be used once, more than once or not at all.

6.   These tests are present in Addenbrooke's cognitive examination.

7.   Asking a patient to interpret proverbs is an appropriate test.

8.   Constructional apraxia and left–right disorientation are localised to this lobe.

9.   Serial sevens tests this cognitive domain.

10. The go–no-go test assesses functions of this lobe.

ASSESSMENT

Theme: Assessment of movement disorders

Options for questions: 11–12

A   Akathisia
B   Athetosis
C   Catalepsy
D   Cataplexy
E   Dystonia
F   Hemiballismus
G   Huntington's disease
H   Myoclonus

For each of the following cases, select the single most likely movement disorder that describes it. Each option may be used once, more than once or not at all.

11. An 80-year-old woman was recovering from left-sided hemiplegia after an intracranial haemorrhage a few weeks ago. She had developed sudden aimless and vigorous movements of her trunk and left arm.

12. A 20-year-old man was admitted after a relapse in his schizophrenia. He was restless, agitated and aggressive on admission. He received 10 mg haloperidol intramuscularly. On day 2, he developed involuntary painful protrusion of his tongue.

Theme: Assessment of psychotic disorders

Options for questions: 13–16

A   Command auditory hallucinations
B   Complex visual hallucinations
C   Delusions of special mission
D   Highly variable delusional content
E   Hypnopompic hallucinations

F   Intermittent depressive symptoms
G   Mood-congruent delusions
H   Passivity experiences
I   Visual impairment

For each of the following diagnoses, select the symptoms and signs as instructed. Each option may be used once, more than once or not at all.

13. Paranoid schizophrenia (select THREE options).

14. Persistent delusional disorder (select THREE options).

15. Charles Bonnet syndrome (select TWO options).

16. Thalamic tumour (select ONE option).

AETIOLOGY

Theme: Risk factors for cognitive disorders

Options for questions: 17–20

A   Anticholinergic drugs
B   Apolipoprotein E_4 gene
C   Diabetes mellitus
D   Electroconvulsive therapy
E   High dietary intake of aluminium

F   Hormone replacement therapy
G   Hypertension
H   Small vessel disease
I   Thiamine deficiency

For each of the following diagnoses, select the single most likely risk factor. Each option may be used once, more than once or not at all.

17. Alzheimer's disease

18. Delirium

19. Korsakoff's syndrome

20. Vascular dementia

DIAGNOSIS

Theme: Sleep disorders and sexual preference disorders

Options for questions: 21–25

A   Ego dystonic sexual orientation
B   Nightmares
C   Paedophilia
D   Sadomasochism

E   Sexual maturation disorder
F   Sleep terrors
G   Somnambulism
H   Voyeurism

For each of the following descriptions, select the single most likely diagnosis. Each option may be used once, more than once or not at all.

21. Tendency to observe people engaging in intimate and sexual behaviours.

22. A sexual preference for children.

23. Uncertainty about gender or sexual orientation causing depression or anxiety.

24. Sexual activity involving inflicting pain.

25. Individual walking in his sleep without awareness, performing motor activities.

Theme: Assessment of psychotic disorders

Options for questions: 26–29

A   Constricted affect, eccentric, poor rapport with others, odd beliefs and suspiciousness for 2 years
B   Does not meet the general criteria for schizophrenia, self-absorbed attitude, social withdrawal, marked apathy, paucity of speech, marked decline in social and occupational performance for over a period of 1 year
C   Delusion or hallucinations must be prominent for 4 weeks
D   Delusions present for 3 months and no persistent hallucinations

E   Flattening or shallowness of affect, aimless or disjointed behaviour, definite thought disorder
F   Met the general criteria for schizophrenia in the past but not now, psychomotor slowing, lack of initiative, poor social performance and poverty of content of speech for at least 12 months
G   Stupor, purposeless motor activity, maintenance of inappropriate postures and rigidity for 2 weeks
H   Two weeks of acute onset of delusions, hallucinations or incoherent speech

For each of the following diagnoses, select the single most likely description from above. Each option may be used once, more than once or not at all.

26. Hebephrenic schizophrenia

27. Catatonic schizophrenia

28. Simple schizophrenia

29. Residual schizophrenia

BASIC PSYCHOLOGICAL PROCESSES

Theme: Learning theories

Options for questions: 30–33

A	Acquisition stage	F	Optimal conditioning
B	Backward conditioning	G	Simultaneous conditioning
C	Generalisation	H	Stimulus discrimination
D	Habituation	I	Trace conditioning
E	Higher-order conditioning		

For each of the following cases, select the single most appropriate description. Each option may be used once, more than once or not at all.

30. Patient was presented with the conditioned stimulus at the same time as the unconditioned stimulus to achieve the conditioned response.

31. Once the patient has made an association with a conditioned stimulus, other similar stimuli can elicit the same response.

32. The patient learnt the association between the conditioned stimulus and the unconditioned stimulus.

33. The interval of time between the presentation of the unconditioned stimulus and the conditioned stimulus should be <0.5 s.

HUMAN PSYCHOLOGICAL DEVELOPMENT

Theme: Reinforcement schedules (programming)

Options for questions: 34–36

A	A response accidentally reinforced by coincidental pairing of response and reinforcement	D	Animal must make an anticipatory response to prevent the punishment
B	An organism changes its behaviour to avoid a painful or noxious stimulus	E	Behaviour engaged in with high frequency can be used to reinforce low-frequency behaviour
C	Animal jumps off an electric grid when the grid is charged	F	Changing behaviour in a deliberate and predetermined way

For each of the following reinforcement schedules, select the single most likely option. Each option may be used once, more than once or not at all.

34. Shaping behaviour

35. Avoidance learning

36. Adventitious reinforcement

DESCRIPTION AND MEASUREMENT

Theme: Measures of memory

Options for questions: 37–41

A	Auditory verbal learning test	F	Recognition memory test
B	California verbal learning test	G	Rey complex figure test
C	Cambridge cognitive examination	H	Rivermead behavioural memory test
D	Doors and people test	I	Wechsler adult intelligence scale – III
E	The MMSE	J	Wechsler memory scale – III

For each of the following descriptions, select the single most appropriate test. Each option may be used once, more than once or not at all.

37. It includes five presentations of a 15-word list (list A), each followed by an attempted recall. This is followed by a second 15-word inter-reference list (list B), followed by recall (list A).

38. It evolved from auditory verbal learning test and attempts to reflect the mult-functional ways in which patients learn or fail to learn verbal material. It has a variety of memory measures such as short- and long-term free recall and recognition, serial learning curve, etc.

39. It was specifically designed to try to detect impairment of everyday memory function by providing test items that resemble activities in everyday life. It has four matched parallel versions.

40. It consists of the presentation of a complicated figure which the patient is asked to copy. The original and copy are then removed and the patient is asked to draw the figure again from memory at varying delayed intervals.

41. It consists of four sections. It was devised to provide comparable measures of visual and verbal memory that test both recall and recognition, do not provide floor or ceiling effects, and include both learning and forgetting measures.

Theme: Measures of premorbid intellectual attainment

Options for questions: 42–45

A	Boston naming test	E	Spot the word test
B	Cambridge contextual reading test	F	Wechsler adult intelligence scale – III
C	National adult reading test (NART)	G	Wechsler test of adult reading
D	Raven's progressive matrices		

For each of the following descriptions, select the single most appropriate test. Each option may be used once, more than once or not at all.

42. This is an oral reading test. It consists of 50 single words. The words are irregular and violate grapheme–phoneme correspondence rules.

43. This test consists of a lexical task. It requires the patient to identify 'real' words from pairs of words or pseudo-words.

44. It is a 50-item word pronunciation test developed to provide an estimate of premorbid intellectual attainment of a person aged 16–89 years. It provides tables of statistical significance for interpreting predicted obtained minus values.

45. It contains some of the NART words embedded in sentences to provide a meaningful context for the patient, e.g. the bride brought a beautiful bouquet.

DESCRIPTIVE PSYCHOPATHOLOGY

Theme: Diagnosis of uncommon syndromes

Options for questions: 46–48

A Blocq's disease
B Briquet's syndrome
C Cotard's syndrome
D Couvade's syndrome

E Diogenes syndrome
F Fregoli's syndrome
G Othello's syndrome

For each of the following cases, select the single most likely diagnosis. Each option may be used once, more than once or not at all.

46. A 41-year-old married woman of previously good health had developed episodes of inability to stand or wait in a normal manner. She often swayed while walking then regained her composure.

47. A 35-year-old man's partner was 30 weeks' pregnant. He presented to his general practitioner with multiple physical symptoms such as nausea, abdominal pain, food craving, toothache. His physical examination revealed no abnormality.

48. A 74-year-old widow presented with complaints of inability to think because she had been dead since her husband died 4 months ago. She also believed that her whole body smelt and therefore her daughter cannot stand next to her.

DYNAMIC PSYCHOPATHOLOGY

Theme: Identification of ego defence mechanisms

Options for questions: 49–52

A Denial
B Displacement
C Identification
D Isolation
E Projection

F Rationalisation
G Reaction formation
H Regression
I Repression
J Sublimation

For each of the following scenarios, select the defence mechanism from the list above that is best illustrated in each scenario. Each option may be used once, more than once or not at all.

49. A 35-year-old man was demoted at his work place because he could not reach the targets. When he returned home, he started shouting at his wife and 8-year-old son.

50. A 20-year-old woman attended your outpatient clinic. She alleged that she was sexually abused when she was 8 years old but she did not remember who the culprit was.

51. A 37-year-old woman who disliked her boss thought that she liked him but felt that he did not like her.

52. A parent who unconsciously resented a child spoils the child with outlandish gifts.

Theme: Identification of ego defence mechanisms

Options for questions: 53–56

A Denial	F Rationalisation
B Displacement	G Reaction formation
C Identification	H Regression
D Isolation	I Repression
E Projection	J Sublimation

For each of the following scenarios, select the defence mechanism from the list above which is best illustrated in each scenario. Each option may be used once, more than once or not at all.

53. A 19-year-old man had temper tantrums when he did not get his way.

54. A 17-year-old male student watched TV instead of studying, saying that the additional study would not do any good anyway.

55. An insecure 22-year-old man joined a fraternity to boost his self-esteem.

56. A 30-year-old traumatised soldier had no recollection of the details of a close brush with death.

History of psychiatry

Theme: Pioneers in psychiatry

Options for questions: 57–59

A Antipsychiatry movement	E Discovered lithium
B Cataplexy	F Electroconvulsive therapy
C Coined the term 'schizophrenia'	G Stress vulnerability model
D Developed IQ test	K Several weeks to several months

For each of the following names, select the single most likely option. Each option may be used once or more than once or none at all.

57. Binet and Simon (1905)

58. David Cooper (1960s)

59. Zubin and Spring (1977)

STIGMA AND CULTURE

Theme: Differential diagnosis of culture-bound syndromes

Options for questions: 60–62

A   Amok
B   Dhat
C   Koro
D   Latah

E   Locura
F   Spell
G   Zar

For each of the following cases, select the single most likely diagnosis. Each option may be used once or more than once or none at all.

60. A 30-year-old Philippino man presented with outbursts of violence, automatism and amnesia of the episode.

61. A 34-year-old Ethiopian man had been shouting and hitting his head against the wall.

62. A 26-year-old man was incoherent, agitated, had auditory and visual hallucinations, and was unpredictable and violent.

Theme: Duration of symptoms necessary for the ICD-10 diagnoses

Options for questions: 63–67

A   4 days
B   7 days
C   2 weeks
D   1 month
E   2 months

F   3 months
G   4 months
H   6 months
I   12 months
J   24 months

For each of the following ICD-10 diagnoses, select the single most appropriate duration of symptoms. Each option may be used once, more than once or not at all.

63. Depression

64. Somatisation

65. Dysthymia

66. Delusional disorder

67. Generalised anxiety disorder

Theme: Disorders of sexual preferences and gender identity disorders

Options for questions: 68–70

A   It is present for a period of 6 months
B   It is present for at least 2 years
C   It is closely associated with sexual arousal and the person removes the clothes after the orgasm
D   Individual wears clothing of the opposite sex in order to be a member of the opposite gender
E   No intention of having sexual intercourse with the person witnessing it
F   Persistent or recurrent urge to watch people engaging in sexual or intimate behaviour
G   The individual desires to live and be accepted as a member of opposite sex by undergoing reassignment surgery

H   The individual wears clothing of the opposite sex to have temporary membership of that gender
I   The person does not have other mental disorders such as schizophrenia or chromosomal abnormalities
J   There is no sexual motivation for the cross-dressing
K   There is a recurrent or persistent desire to expose the genitalia to strangers

For each of the following cases, select the most appropriate options according to further instructions. Each option may be used once, more than once or not at all.

68.   Role transvestism (select **TWO** options).

69.   Transsexualism (select **THREE** options).

70.   Exhibitionism (select **THREE** options).

Answers: EMIs

1. A Acknowledging emotions

If a doctor comments on the patient's emotions and acknowledges it, it is called acknowledging the emotions.

2. B Compound question

Such questioning style is considered to be one of the obstructive interventions in the psychiatric interview.

3. C Dismissal

This style is also called minimisation. Encouragement is a type of supportive intervention.

4. D Encouragement

Appropriate use of open and closed questions is very important to gather more information. There are some supportive and obstructive interventions in carrying out the psychiatric interview.

5. E Judgemental

This is a type of obstructive intervention.

6. D Clock-drawing test

The Addenbrooke's cognitive examination is now widely used as a more sensitive measure of cognitive ability. It takes around 15 minutes to administer and is marked out of 100. It includes more detailed cognitive tests including frontal lobe tests.

7. F Frontal lobe

There are various frontal lobe tests, some of which include interpretation of proverbs, cognitive estimates, verbal fluency and motor fluency. In proverb interpretation, the patient is asked the meaning of common proverbs such as 'too many cooks spoil the broth'. The go–no-go test is another frontal lobe test in which the patient is asked to respond to a cue; it tests sustained attention. Examples include asking the patient to lift a finger on hearing a tapping sound and subsequently dropping it after hearing two tapping sounds.

8. I Parietal lobe

The parietal lobe has a number of functions including left–right orientation. Test for left–right confusion ask the patient to show his or her right and then the left hand. If this is correctly performed, ask the patient to touch his or her left ear with the right hand, and vice versa. Constructional apraxia can be demonstrated by asking the patient to copy interlocking pentagons.

9. C Attention and concentration

Serial sevens are present in both the MMSE and Addenbrooke's examination as a test on attention and concentration. The patient is asked to subtract 7 from 100 and this is done a total of 5 times, giving a score out of five.

10. F Frontal lobe

There are various frontal lobe tests, some of which include interpretation of proverbs, cognitive estimates, verbal fluency and motor fluency. In proverb interpretation the patient is asked the meaning of common proverbs such as 'too many cooks spoil the broth'. The go–no-go test is another frontal lobe test in which the patient is asked to respond to a cue; it tests sustained attention. Examples include asking the patient to lift a finger on hearing a tapping sound and subsequently dropping it after hearing two tapping sounds.

11. F Hemiballismus

This is called hemiballism, and includes violent swinging movements of one side, usually caused by infarction or haemorrhage in the contralateral subthalamic nucleus.

12. E Dystonia

Acute dytonias occur within 5 days of exposure, or slightly closer, in 90% of instances. Dystonias affect up to a third of patients on high-potency antipsychotics but fewer on low-potency drugs. They respond readily to anticholinergic drugs.

13. A, C, H Command auditory hallucinations. Delusions of special mission. Passivity experiences

In paranoid schizophrenia, hallucinations and delusions are prominent and the personality is relatively well preserved.

14. C, D, F Delusions of special mission. Highly variable delusional content. Intermittent depressive symptoms

Persistent delusional disorder is characterised by one or more non-bizarre delusions or a delusional system. Duration criteria for the ICD-10 are 3 months, whereas those for the DSM-IV are only 1 month.

15. B, I Complex visual hallucinations. Visual impairment

The Charles Bonnet syndrome is characterised by formed, complex, persistent, repetitive and stereotyped visual hallucinations, recognised by that patient as not real without any other hallucinations or delusions.

16. E Hypnopompic hallucination

Thalamic tumours have been reported to show early and severe dementia, which runs a rapid course.

17. B Apolipoprotein E4 gene

Apolipoprotein E polymorphism (ApoE, alleles E_2, E_3, E_4) has been identified as a main genetic risk factor for Alzheimer's disease (AD) in all age groups. It has been demonstrated that E4 alleles occur more commonly in AD and have a dose-dependent effect and accelerate the time of onset. The ApoE$_2$ allele appears to confer some protection against the development of AD, but its mechanism of action remains unknown. It should be emphasised that ApoE allele testing is not part of routine clinical practice. They have been identified on the *APP* gene (chromosome 21), presenilin-1 gene (chromosome 14) and presenilin-2 gene (chromosome 1).

18. A Anticholinergic drugs

Delirium occurs particularly in association with increasing age, anxiety, sensory under- or over-stimulation, drug dependence and brain damage of all types. It also occurs in association with drug intoxication or withdrawal of alcohol, the drugs involved being anticholinergics, anxiolytics, hypnotics and anticonvulsants. Urinary tract infection, septicaemia, endocarditis and pneumonia are common causes of delirium.

19. I Thiamine deficiency

Chronic alcohol abuse associated with thiamine deficiency is the most frequent cause of Korsakoff's syndrome. Petechial haemorrhages with astrocyte degeneration are found in the mammillary bodies, the region of the third ventricle, the periaqueductal grey matter, pons and medial dorsal thalamic nuclei.

20. G Hypertension

In addition, multiple strokes and subdural haematomas are predominant causes of vascular dementia.

21. H Voyeurism

This is a disorder of sexual preference. The duration of symptoms ought to be present for a period of 6 months. There is a persistent or recurrent desire to observe others indulging in intimate behaviours without having any desire to perform sexual intercourse with the observed.

22. C Paedophilia

This is disorder of sexual preference. The minimum duration of symptoms is for 6 months. There is a persistent or predominant desire to indulge in sexual activity with a prepubescent child. The person indulging in such behaviour ought to be 16 years and at least 5 years older than the child.

23. E Sexual maturation disorder

The person has confusion about sexual orientation. It occurs mostly in people who are not certain about their orientation. For them finding their orientation is challenging.

24. D Sadomasochism

This is a disorder of sexual preference.

25. G Somnambulism

This is commonly known as sleepwalking. The person is not even aware of it, and sometimes performs some tasks during that phase. People have been reported driving during these episodes. Night terrors usually occur at an early age. The person wakes up screaming and shouting, and later has no recollection of it.

26. E Flattening or shallowness of affect, aimless or disjointed behaviour, definite thought disorder

The onset of hebephrenic schizophrenia is usually in the late teens and interferes with the thought processes. There is sustained swallowing and inappropriateness of affect. The behaviour is noted to be aimless and disjointed. There is a formal thought disorder.

27. G Stupor, purposeless motor activity, maintenance of inappropriate postures and rigidity for 2 weeks

The general criteria for schizophrenia are met but there are additional symptoms present for at least 2 weeks which consist of stupor, increased motor activity and posturing, negativism and command automatisms.

28. B Does not meet the general criteria for schizophrenia, self-absorbed attitude, social withdrawal, marked apathy, paucity of speech, marked decline in social and occupational performance for over a period of 1 year

Simple schizophrenia does not fulfil the general criteria for schizophrenia. For a year there will have been symptoms of social withdrawal, increased negative symptoms such as apathy and paucity of speech. There is a noted academic decline.

29. F Met the general criteria for schizophrenia in the past but not now, psychomotor slowing, lack of initiative, poor social performance and poverty of content of speech for at least 12 months

Residual schizophrenia does not meet the general criteria of schizophrenia at the time of assessment but must have met the criteria at some point. There are 12 months of negative symptoms. It includes psychomotor slowing, blunting of affect, lack of initiative, poor non-verbal communication and poor social performance or self-care.

30. G Simultaneous conditioning

In the study of learning and conditioning, the work by Pavlov observed the process of classic conditioning. Here, through repeated association of an unconditioned stimulus with a conditioned stimulus, a conditioned response is achieved. His work was demonstrated by observation of a dog salivating to food then pairing the stimulus of food, with the sound of the bell, so that the dog was conditioned to salivate to the sound of the bell over time.

31. C Generalisation

The responses occur once the patient has made an association with a conditioned stimulus; other similar stimuli can elicit the same response.

32. A Acquisition stage

This is a stage is in which the participant learns the association between the conditioned stimulus and the unconditioned stimulus.

33. F Optimal conditioning

This is the interval of time between the presentation of the unconditioned stimulus and the conditioned stimulus; it should be <0.5 seconds. Simultaneous conditioning is when the participant is presented with the conditioned stimulus at the same time as the unconditioned stimulus to achieve the conditioned response.

34. F Changing behaviour in a deliberate and predetermined way

Shaping behaviour means changing behaviour in a deliberate and predetermined manner. It is also called successive approximation.

35. D Animal must make an anticipatory response to prevent the punishment

An organism changes its behaviour to avoid a painful or noxious stimulus – aversive control. When an animal jumps off an electric grid, it is called escape learning.

36. A A response accidentally reinforced by coincidental pairing of response and reinforcement

Behaviour engaged with high frequency can be used to reinforce low-frequency behaviour. It is called Premack's principle.

37. A Auditory verbal learning test

there are various tests used in research and practice to test memory and learning. One of the most commonly used test to test word learning is an auditory verbal learning test. In this test, delayed recall and recognition are also tested.

38. B California verbal learning test

This is the advanced version. It includes things tested in an auditory verbal learning test and also some common things such as observing a person while shopping.

39. H Rivermead behavioural memory test

This is a four-match parallel version in which the effects of clinical intervention and progression of disease can be measured or determined. The extended Rivermead behavioural memory test (RBMT) is useful in separating out those individuals who scored at the upper range of the original RBMT.

40. G Rey complex figure test

This has useful normative data for those up to the age of 93 years. Its test–re-test reliability was reported as 0.76 for immediate recall and 0.89 for delayed recall.

41. D Doors and people test

The door and people test has got four sections. In the door test, a person has to recognise single doors against the distracters, which are competing. In the shape test, a person has to reproduce the different diagrams from memory. The name test is a verbal recognition test. In the people test, a person needs to relate and learn from different photographs and names.

42. C National adult reading test (NART)

Various tests are used to find out a person's premorbid intelligence. One of the tests used is called the NART. In this test, a person is asked to pronounce infrequent words. It usually goes with a patient's educational level. It contains 50 items. It has been suggested that it is inappropriate to estimate premorbid ability in Korsakoff's syndrome using the NART.

43. E Spot the word test

This is mainly limited to research applications.

In the word test a person has to recognise a true word or real word from a series of word that can be pseudo-words. At the moment it is just a research tool.

44. G Wechsler test of adult reading

It is co-normed with the WAIS-III and the Wechsler memory scale III (WMS-III). Therefore, one can directly compare the Wechsler test of adult reading's predicted scores with those from WAIS-III and WMS-III.

45. B Cambridge contextual reading test

unfortunately, the Cambridge contextual reading test (CCRT) has not been normed against current measures of intelligence (e.g. WAIS-III), so it is not possible to readily use the CCRT to estimate premorbid attainments.

46. A Blocq's disease

This is also called astasia–abasia. It is characterised by the inability to walk or stand in a normal way. The gait is bizarre and does not suggest any organic brain lesion. The patient is often noticed to be swaying and falling, with recovery at the last moment. It is considered a conversion/dissociative symptom.

47. D Couvade's syndrome

This is characterised by an experience of self in which a spouse/partner complains of obstetric symptoms during his partner's pregnancy and parturition. The condition usually arises in the second and third trimesters. It also consists of nausea, abdominal pain, toothache, food cravings and preoccupation with the spouse/partner's condition. The person is not delusional because he does not believe that he is pregnant. It is akin to a conversion disorder in which his anxieties about his wife/partner's pregnancy are converted into physical symptoms.

48. C Cotard's syndrome

This is characterised by a delusion in which a person believes that he or she is dead. It may be accompanied by other nihilistic delusions that he or she is rotting, smell malodorous or parts of the body do not exist.

49. B Displacement

This means diverting emotional feelings (usually anger) from their original source to a substitute target. Here the original source of anger was the work place and substitute targets were the wife and son.

50. I Repression

This means keeping distressing thoughts and feelings buried in the unconscious. Memories of sexual abuse are distressing, and therefore buried in the unconscious (motivated forgetting).

51. E Projection

This means attributing one's own thoughts, feelings or motives to another woman who dislikes her boss (her own feelings) or a boss who dislikes her (projection).

52. G Reaction formation

This means behaving in a way that is exactly the opposite of one's true feelings: parent resents the child (true feelings) or outlandish gifts (opposite behaviour).

53. H Regression

This is a reversion to immature patterns of behaviour. A temper tantrum is an immature behaviour for an adult.

54. F Rationalisation

This means creating false but plausible excuses to justify unacceptable behaviour such as watching TV (unacceptable behaviour) or why additional study would not do any good (false excuse).

55. C Identification

This means bolstering self-esteem by forming an imaginary or real alliance with some person or group, e.g. joining a fraternity (a real alliance with a group).

56. I Repression

This means keeping distressing thoughts and feelings buried in the unconscious. A memory of a close brush with death is distressing and therefore forgotten (buried in the unconscious, motivated forgetting).

57. D Developed IQ test

Binet and Simon developed their first IQ test in 1905.

58. A Antipsychiatry movement

David Cooper revived the antipsychiatry movement in 1960s. He was a committed Marxist and saw schizophrenia as a form of social repression.

59. B Cataplexy

Henneberg coined the term 'cataplexy' in 1916.

60. D Amok

This is a dissociative state in men after a period of brooding and then an outburst of violence, aggression or homicidal behaviour. The episode is also accompanied by automatism and amnesia, and there is a return to the premorbid state after the episode finishes. It was originally found in Malaysia, but is also recorded in Laos, the Philippines, Polynesia, Papua New Guinea, Puerto Rico and among the Navajo.

61. G Zar

This is a condition in which a person believes that he or she is possessed by spirits. It may present as a dissociative episode and include singing, shouting, laughing, crying and head banging. The patient may show apathy, withdrawal, or refusal to eat or do daily tasks. The patient may develop a relationship with the possessing spirit.

62. F Spell

This is a trance state in which a person communicates with deceased relatives or spirits. It occurs among African–Americans and European Americans from South America.

63. C 2 weeks

A minimum duration of 2 weeks is required to make a diagnosis of obsessive–compulsive disorder which is characterised by obsessions (thoughts, ruminations, impulses, 'phobias'), compulsive rituals, abnormal slowness, anxiety, depression and depersonalisation.

64. J 24 months

A minimum duration of 24 months is required to diagnose somatisation disorder.

65. J 24 months

A minimum duration of 24 months is required to a diagnose dysthymia.

66. F 3 months

A minimum duration of 3 months is required to diagnose delusional disorder.

67. K Several weeks to several months

The patient must suffer from primary anxiety symptoms most days for at least several weeks to several months at a time. According to the ICD-10, the timescale for symptoms of depression is 2 weeks, for dysthymia or cyclothymia 2 years, for schizophrenia 4 weeks according to the ICD-10 and 6 months per the DSM-IV, for mania 7 days, for hypomani 4 days and for hypochondriacal disorder 6 months

68. G, H The individual desires to live and be accepted as a member of the opposite sex by undergoing reassignment surgery. The individual wears clothing of the opposite sex to have temporary membership of that gender

Dual-role transvestism is a gender identity disorder. There is a desire for temporary membership of the opposite gender. There is no sexual arousal associated with cross-dressing.

69. B, G, I It is present for at least 2 years. The individual desires to live and be accepted as a member of the opposite sex by undergoing reassignment surgery. The person does not have other mental disorders such as schizophrenia or chromosomal abnormalities

Transsexualism is a gender identity disorder. The desire is to be accepted as a member of the opposite sex. Reassignment surgery is the pinnacle for the change of role and membership of the opposite gender. It must be present for a period of at least 2 years.

70. A, E, K It is present for a period of 6 months. No intention of having sexual intercourse with the person witnessing it. There is a recurrent or persistent desire to expose the genitalia to strangers

Exhibitionism is a disorder of sexual preference. It should be present for at least 6 months. It is one of the most common disorders of sexual preference, present predominantly in the male gender. There is a desire to show the genitalia to a specific age group, followed by masturbation. There is no desire for sexual intercourse with the witness.

Chapter 4

Test questions: 4

Questions: EMIs

HISTORY AND MENTAL STATE EXAMINATION

Theme: Assessment of abnormal movements

Options for questions: 1–5

A	Echolalia		F	*Mitgehen*
B	Echopraxia		G	*Mitmachen*
C	*Gegenhalten*		H	Negativism
D	Logoclonia		I	Palilalia
E	Mannerism		J	Stereotypies

For each of the following cases, select the single most likely abnormal movement or psychopathology that best describes it. Each option may be used once, more than once or not at all.

1. A 27-year-old patient with a psychotic disorder, who has been stable for 2 years, attended the outpatient clinic for a review. He was noticed to be carrying out purposeless motor acts repetitively and with a high degree of uniformity.

2. A 23-year-old patient with a psychotic disorder attended the outpatient clinic for review. During examination he opposed all passive movements with the same force as was applied.

3. A 75-year-old woman attended the outpatient clinic for a review. She was instructed to resist all movements but allowed the clinician to put her body in any position without any resistance.

4. A 69-year-old patient with Alzheimer's disease attended the outpatient clinic for a review. During examination, she was asked to repeat 'I am well today' but said 'I am well today-ay-ay-ay-ay'.

5. A 77-year-old patient with Alzheimer's disease attended the outpatient clinic for a review. During examination, she was asked to repeat 'I am well today' but kept repeating 'today' with increasing frequency.

COGNITIVE ASSESSMENT

Theme: Disorders of speech

Options for questions: 6–9

A   Broca's aphasia
B   Conduction aphasia
C   Global aphasia
D   Nominal aphasia

E   Pure word blindness
F   Transcortical motor aphasia
G   Transcortical sensory aphasia
H   Wernicke's aphasia

For each of the following cases, select the single most likely speech disorder. Each option may be used once, more than once or not at all.

6.   A 37-year-old man's speech has repetition and comprehension that are intact but fluency and naming are lost.

7.   In a 46-year-old man with aphasia, repetition, comprehension and naming are lost and only fluency is intact

8.   In a 59-year-old woman with aphasia, fluency, repetition and naming are lost and only comprehension is intact.

9.   In a 71-year-old woman with aphasia, the speech is telegraphic.

NEUROLOGICAL EXAMINATION

Theme: Assessment of apraxias

Options for questions: 10–14

A   Apraxia of gait
B   Apraxia of speech
C   Buccofacial apraxia
D   Constructional apraxia

E   Dressing apraxia
F   Ideational apraxia
G   Ideomotor apraxia
H   Limb kinetic apraxia

For each of the following cases, select the single most likely apraxia. Each option may be used once, more than once or not at all.

10.   A 72-year-old man had memory difficulties with gradual and progressive deterioration. He was unable to copy interlocking pentagons in the MMSE.

11.   An 81-year-old woman found it difficult to prepare a cup of tea because she was unable to perform a multiple-step task.

12.   An 80-year-old man was brought by his daughter to an outpatient appointment. When he was given a screwdriver, he started writing with it as if it was a pen.

13.   An 83-year-old woman could not perform skilled movements involving the lips, mouth and tongue, e.g. whistling or coughing.

14.   A 66-year-old patient attended the accident and emergency department with complaints of urinary incontinence and cognitive impairment, and was not able to walk or stand without support.

ASSESSMENT

Theme: Diagnosis of neurotic disorders

Options for questions: 15–19

A	Acute stress reaction	F	Obsessive–compulsive disorder
B	Adjustment disorder	G	Panic disorder
C	Agoraphobia	H	Post-traumatic stress disorder
D	Body dysmorphophobic disorder	I	Social phobia
E	Generalised anxiety disorder	J	Specific phobia

For each of the following cases, select the single most likely diagnosis. Each option may be used once, more than once or not at all.

15. A 28-year-old man had cold chills and trembling when in crowds and public places.

16. A 32-year-old woman had hot flushes, palpitations, blushing and urgency when eating out in a busy restaurant with a small group of friends.

17. A 36-year-old woman had sweating and a dry mouth along with fear on seeing a spider crawling in the living area.

18. After a road traffic accident, a 44-year-old woman experienced disorientation, agitation and excessive crying that persisted for 2 days.

19. A 52-year-old man was refused asylum. He had appealed against it but began to experience mild depression 3 weeks after the decision by the immigration department.

Theme: Assessment of memory

Options for questions: 20–22

A	Confabulation	E	Registration
B	Jamais-vu	F	Remembering
C	Recognition	G	Retrieval
D	Recollection	H	Retrospective falsification

For each of the following, select the single most likely option from above that best describes it. Each option may be used once, more than once or not at all.

20. It is a process that involves reintegration of a complete event from a variety of components.

21. It consists of modification of memories in terms of one's general attitudes.

22. It is the feeling of familiarity that normally occurs with previously experienced events. However, it is absent when the event is experienced a second time.

AETIOLOGY

Theme: Assessment of risk factors

Options for questions: 23–25

A   Antacid use
B   Being involved in an accident 8 months ago
C   Having human leukocyte antigen (HLA)-B27 factor in the blood
D   Having been raped 4 months ago
E   History of rape in childhood
F   Reduced vision following a cataract operation
G   Regular use of laxatives

For each of the following cases, select the single most likely risk factor. Each option may be used once, more than once or not at all.

23. An 81-year-old man with good memory experiences visual hallucinations.

24. A 34-year-old single woman presented with chronic feeling of emptiness, affective instability, intense frequent changes in relationships and frequent self-harm acts.

25. A 30-year-old single woman experienced low moods, anger, recurrent nightmares and flashbacks, and was startled easily.

DIAGNOSIS

Theme: Diagnosis of mood disorders

Options for questions: 26–27

A   Grief reaction
B   Mild depressive episode with somatic syndrome
C   Moderate depressive episode with somatic syndrome
D   Pathological grief reaction
E   Postnatal depression
F   Puerperal psychosis
G   Severe depressive episode with psychotic symptoms
H   Severe depressive episode without psychotic symptoms

For each of the following cases, select the single most likely diagnosis. Each option may be used once, more than once or not at all.

26. An 81-year-old widower presented 4 months after his wife's unexpected death with tearfulness, poor appetite, weight loss, sleep disturbance and loss of interest in life. At times, he could hear his dead wife calling out his name and asking him to join her. He did not wish to part with any of her belongings.

27. A 59-year-old factory worker who was made redundant 2 months ago presented with depressed mood, loss of appetite, loss of weight of 8 kg, excessive tiredness, early morning waking and loss of interest in life. He complained of hearing his supervisor's voice telling him he was completely useless and did not deserve to live.

Theme: Diagnosis of uncommon syndromes

Options for questions: 28–30

A   Blocq's disease
B   Briquet's syndrome
C   Cotard's syndrome
D   Couvade's syndrome
E   Diogenes syndrome
F   Fregoli's syndrome
G   Othello's syndrome

For each of the following cases, select the single most likely diagnosis. Each option may be used once, more than once or not at all.

28. A 78-year-old retired company director lives on his own since his wife died a few years ago. He has no previous history of any mental disorder. His children noticed that he had become socially reclusive and never visited them since their mother's death. They found him living in total squalor and surrounded by rubbish. They also noticed that the house was infested with worms and rodents. However, he refused any help because he was happy with himself and did not see anything wrong with his house.

29. A 30-year-old married woman presented herself to the accident and emergency department complaining bitterly about her brother. She believed that he could change his appearance, hair-style, clothes, and even his sex whenever he desired to spy on her. She had fallen out with him about 6 months ago.

30. A 45-year-old previously married woman with no past psychiatric history started accusing her husband of a recent extramarital affair. Her husband told her repeatedly and categorically that he was not unfaithful to her but she would not accept his words. She employed a private detective agency to follow his movements and activities.

HUMAN PSYCHOLOGICAL DEVELOPMENT

Theme: Jean Piaget's stages of cognitive development

Options for questions: 31–34

A   Abstract reasoning
B   Conservation
C   Egocentricity
D   Hypothetico-inductive reasoning
E   Operational thought
F   Reversibility
G   Schema of permanent object
H   Semiotic function
I   Symbolisation
J   Syncretic reasoning

For each of the following Piaget's stages of cognitive development, select the most appropriate achievement according to further instructions. Each option may be used once, more than once or not at all.

31. Sensorimotor stage (birth to 2 years) (select TWO options).

32. Preoperational stage (2–7 years) (select TWO options).

33. Concrete operational stage (7–11 years) (select THREE options).

34. Stage of formal operations (11 to early adolescence) (select ONE option).

SOCIAL PSYCHOLOGY

Theme: Parenting styles

Options for questions: 35–38

A	Authoritarian	F	Combination of permissive and hostile
B	Authoritative	G	Combination of permissive and loving
C	Combination of authoritarian and hostile	H	Hostile
D	Combination of authoritarian and loving	I	Loving
E	Combination of authoritarian and permissive	J	Permissive

For each of the following descriptions, select the single most appropriate parenting style. Each option may be used once, more than once or not at all.

35. Parents treat their child as equal.

36. Parents make unrealistic demands and they punish their child to control the behaviour.

37. Parents make few demands and they provide less guidance.

38. A child tries to over-achieve to please the parents.

DESCRIPTION AND MEASUREMENT

Theme: Assessment of personality disorders

Options for questions: 39–43

A	Hare Levenson self-report psychopathy scales	F	Personality assessment schedule
B	Hare psychopathy checklist – revised	G	Personality disorder questionnaire
C	International personality disorders examination	H	Schedule of non-adaptive and adaptive personality
D	Millon clinical multiaxial inventory	I	Structured clinical interview for DSM-IV axis II personality disorders
E	Neuroticism, extroversion, openness – personality inventory	J	Structured clinical interview for DSM-IV personality

For each of the following descriptions, select the single most appropriate test. Each option may be used once, more than once or not at all.

39. This instrument is a self-administered questionnaire of 175 items. It takes 25 minutes to complete and is analysed by computers.

40. This instrument generates diagnosis for both the ICD-10 and the DSM-IV. It requires either the participant or the informant or both to provide information on 24 personality traits.

41. This instrument is the most popular personality questionnaire. It consists of 250 self-rating items on a 5-point Likert scale.

42. The instrument is a semi-structured clinical interview with 101 questions in a thematic version and 107 questions in a disorder-by-disorder version.

43. This instrument is a screening questionnaire for the ICD-10 and DSM-IV versions, which can be used to identify people who are unlikely to have a personality disorder.

DESCRIPTIVE PSYCHOPATHOLOGY

Theme: Assessment of thought disorders

Options for questions: 44–46

A	Circumstantiality	E	Perseveration
B	Derailment	F	Tangentiality
C	Desultory thinking	G	Thought blocking
D	Drivelling thinking		

For each of the following cases, select the single most likely psychopathology. Each option may be used once, more than once or not at all.

44. When a 63-year-old man was asked where he lived as a child he replied, 'Arsenal is my favourite football team'.

45. A 77-year-old man was asked to name the present Prime Minister; he repeated, 'David Cameron, David Cameron' despite being asked different questions.

46. A 23-year-old man was asked to explain why he was referred to your clinic. He gave a long answer. This occurs when thinking proceeds slowly with many unnecessary and trivial details but finally the point is reached.

Theme: Disorders of memory

Options for questions: 47–50

A	Confabulation	F	Recollection
B	Déjà-vu	G	Registration
C	Dissociative amnesia	H	Retrieval
D	Jamais-vu	I	Retrospective falsification
E	Recognition	J	Semantic memory

For each of the following descriptions, select the options as instructed. Each option may be used once, more than once or not at all.

47. This is responsible for a permanent storage of representational knowledge of facts, concepts, objects and people, as well as words and their meaning (select ONE option)

48. It manifests itself as the filling in of gaps in memory by imagined or untrue experiences that have no basis in fact (select ONE option).

49. These are required for long-term memory (select THREE options).

50. This is a sensation that a situation or event is unfamiliar, even though it has been experienced before (select ONE option).

DYNAMIC PSYCHOPATHOLOGY

Theme: Structure of personality

Options for questions: 51–53

A   Moral component of personality, emerges at 1–2 years of age, operates at all three levels of awareness

B   Moral component of personality, emerges at 3–5 years of age, operates at all three levels of awareness

C   Moral component of personality, emerges at 3–5 years of age, operates at unconscious and preconscious levels only

D   Operates according to the pleasure principle, demands immediate gratification of its urges, engages in primary process thinking, which is fantasy oriented, operates at all three levels of awareness

E   Operates according to the pleasure principle, demands immediate gratification of its urges, and engages in primary process thinking, which is oriented towards problem solving, operates entirely at unconscious level

F   Operates according to the pleasure principle, demands immediate gratification of its urges, and engages in primary process thinking, which is fantasy oriented, operates entirely at unconscious level

G   Operates according to the reality principle, delays the gratification, engages in secondary process thinking, which is oriented towards problem solving, operates at all three levels of awareness

For each of the following, select the single most likely description. Each option may be used once, more than once or not at all.

51. Id

52. Ego

53. Super-ego

Theme: Freud's stages of psychosexual development

Options for questions: 54–58

A   0–1 year of age

B   2–3 years of age

C   4–5 years of age

D   6–12 years of age

E   Puberty onwards

For each of the following stages of development, select the most appropriate age group from the list above. Each option may be used once, more than once or not at all.

54. During this stage there is suppression of the child's sexuality.

55. Fixation at this stage can lead to obsessions and compulsion in later life.

56. Young girls feel hostile towards their mother because they blame her for their anatomical deficiency of not having a penis.

57. There is channelling of sexual energy towards peers of the other sex.

58. Fixation at this stage can lead to excessive smoking in later life.

Theme: Diagnosis of culture-bound syndromes

Options for questions: 59–62

A	Amok	E	Latah
B	Brain fag	F	Locura
C	Dhat	G	Pa-leng
D	Koro	H	Piblokoto

For each of the following cases, select the single most likely diagnosis. Each option may be used once, more than once or not at all.

59. A 32-year-old Malaysian man went into a dissociative state, followed by an outburst of violent and aggressive behaviour.

60. A 25-year-old young Indian man felt that he was losing his semen in his urine, and felt weak and exhausted.

61. A 40-year-old Eskimo woman went into an acute state of excitement followed by seizures or coma.

62. A 30-year-old Chinese man displayed excessive fear of cold for no apparent reason.

NEUROLOGICAL EXAMINATION

Theme: Diagnosis of neuropsychiatric disorders

Options for questions: 63–66

A	Angular gyrus syndrome	E	Gilles de la Tourette's syndrome
B	Anton's syndrome	F	Klüver–Bucy syndrome
C	Balint's syndrome	G	Korsakoff's syndrome
D	Ganser's syndrome	H	Ramsay Hunt syndrome

For each of the following cases, select the single most likely diagnosis. Each option may be used once, more than once or not at all.

63. A 45-year-old man presented with clouding of consciousness with disorientation to time, place and person, and auditory and visual hallucinations. He had recently sustained a head injury. On the Mental State Examination, when asked what the capital of UK was, he replied Birmingham. When he was asked to add 3 and 3, he replied 7. On recovery from his episode, he had complete amnesia.

64. A 29-year-old man presented with an excessive sex drive, putting inanimate objects into his mouth, and attempting to derive sexual gratification by using toys. He was affected by herpes encephalitis.

65. A 31-year-old man presented with unilateral facial paralysis, dry eye, hearing loss, red painful rash, and blisters in the ears and mouth.

66. A 26-year-old man presented with multiple waxing and waning motor and vocal tics. He exhibited echolalia and coprophagia. He was recently also concerned about aggressive thoughts, forced touching, fear of self-harm, cleanliness and hygiene.

DIAGNOSIS

Theme: Diagnosis of childhood and adolescent disorders

Options for questions: 67–71

A   Conduct disorder
B   Disorders of social functioning with onset specific to childhood and adolescence
C   Emotional disorders with onset specific to childhood
D   Hyperkinetic disorder
E   Mixed disorders of conduct and emotions
F   Oppositional defiant disorder
G   Other behavioural disorder and emotional disorders with onset usually occurring in childhood and adolescence
H   Pervasive development disorders
I   Specific development disorders of scholastic skills
J   Specific development disorder of mental function
K   Tic disorders

For each of the following cases, select the single most likely disorder according to the ICD-10. Each option may be used once, more than once or not at all.

67.   A 5-year-old girl was brought in who had a persistent fear of strangers. She clings on to her mother every time a visitor comes to their house. She refuses to go to her new school.

68.   A 5-year-old boy presented with frequent eye blinking and facial grimacing for the past few months. He is of normal intelligence.

69.   A 7-year-old boy presented with intense restlessness, jumping and running into things. His behaviour was considered intolerable at school. He has been disruptive and inattentive in his class.

70.   A 10-year-old boy presented with a history of persistently aggressive, antisocial and defiant behaviour. He got upset very easily. He had a period of marked depression with feelings of hopelessness.

71.   A 6-year-old girl presented with an excessive fear of crowded places and refusal to go shopping with her mother. She had no problem going to her local shops. She went with her parents to visit her grandparents by car and enjoyed her visit.

Answers: EMIs

1. J Stereotypies

A stereotyped movement is a repetitive non-goal-directed action that is carried out in a uniform way. A stereotypy may be a simple movement or repeated utterance. In a verbal stereotypy, the content may be understandable; it may be produced spontaneously or be set off by a question. In contrast mannerisms are normal goal-directed activities but are odd in appearance or out of context.

2. C *Gegenhalten*

Some patients with catatonia oppose all passive movements with some degree of force, as applied by the examiner, called gegenhalten. Often this is not evident when the passive movements are carried out very gently. Negativism can be regarded as an accentuation of opposition.

3. G *Mitmachen*

In mitmachen, the body can be put into any position without any resistance on the part of the patient, although the patient is instructed to resist all movements. Once the examiner lets go of the body part that has been moved, it return to the resting position. *Mitgehen* can be regarded as an extreme form of cooperation, i.e. mitmachen, as the patient moves the body in the direction of the slightest pressure on the part of the examiner.

4. D Logoclonia

This is a special form of perseveration in which the last syllable of the word is repeated.

5. I Palilalia

This is a special form of perseveration in which the patient repeats the perseverated word with increasing frequency.

6. F Transcortical motor aphasia

In transcortical motor aphasia, repetition and comprehension are intact but fluency and naming are lost.

7. H Wernicke's aphasia

Comprehension depends on an intact Wernicke's area and its further connections with association cortex and sensory input. In Wernicke's aphasia, fluency is intact but repetition, comprehension and naming are lost. Comprehension is lost for both spoken and written language. Language is fluent but highly paraphasic, and sometimes neologism and circumlocution also occur, so it is also called jargon aphasia.

8. A Broca's aphasia

Aphasia is a problem of language reception, production and processing. Most of the time aphasia is organic. Fluency depends on an intact Broca's area and its forward connections. A defect in naming the objects is called anomia which accompanies any aphasia to various degrees. In Broca's motor aphasia, fluency, repetition and naming are lost but comprehension is intact.

Sound is transmitted through the ears to Wernicke's area and the auditory association cortex. Arcuate fasciculus connects Wernicke's area to Broca's area, which is considered to be a higher motor area of language production. Signals from Broca's area are transmitted to the motor area to coordinate the delivery of language via the tongue, lips and vocal folds.

9. A Broca's aphasia

Telegraphic speech is seen in Broca's aphasia. It is the use of simple sentences/words that convey important meaning, although with omission of appropriate grammatical usage. Telegraphic speech is seen in children who are acquiring language ability, usually between the ages of 18 and 24 months.

10. D Constructional apraxia

The deficits in skilled movements are termed 'apraxia'. Constructional apraxia is the inability to construct elements to a meaningful whole.

11. F Ideational apraxia

This occurs when the individual components of a sequence of skilled acts can be performed in isolation, but the entire series cannot be organised and executed as a whole.

12. G Ideomotor apraxia

This is the inability to perform an isolated motor act on command, despite preserved comprehension, strength and spontaneous performance of the same act.

13. C Buccofacial apraxia

This is an inability to coordinate and carry out lip and facial movements, e.g. licking lips, whistling.

14. A Apraxia of gait

In normal pressure hydrocephalus, there is a triad of gait apraxia, urinary incontinence and reversible dementia.

15. C Agoraphobia

This is a subcategory of the phobic anxiety disorders in the broad category of neurotic, stress-related and somatoform disorders.

16. I Social phobia

This is characterised by fear of embarrassing oneself, accompanied by autonomic arousal symptoms and also the emotional distress caused by the symptoms themselves. It happens while eating or speaking in public or in small meetings such as parties or even in the classroom.

17. J Specific phobia

They are phobias of inanimate or animate objects. These are characterised by a marked fear of the object, along with autonomic arousal symptoms followed by significant emotional distress.

18. A Acute stress reaction

Acute stress reaction is a disorder that is time limited and manifests as a result of a mental and psychological stressor. There are symptoms of autonomic arousal symptoms. It does not fulfil the criteria of phobic anxiety disorders and is not due to hyperthyroidism, organic mental disorder or psychoactive substance-related issues. There is apparent disorientation, narrowing of attention or inappropriate overactivity. The symptoms appear within minutes of the stressful event and remit from 8 hours post-incident up to 72 hours. Individual predisposition and coping mechanisms play an important role in the incidence and severity of an acute stress reaction.

19. B Adjustment disorder

In adjustment disorders, the onset of symptoms occurs within a month of exposure to a stressor or a significant life change. The symptoms usually last up to 6 months and rarely exceed this limit, except in cases of prolonged depressive reaction. If the symptoms exceed 6 months, the diagnosis should be revised depending on the clinical presentation. Individual predisposition plays an important role in clinical presentation of an adjustment disorder.

20. D Recollection

This is a part of scene memory and is considered to be partly true and partly false.

21. B Jamais-vu

This is the knowledge that an event has been experienced before but is not currently associated with the appropriate feeling of familiarity.

22. H Retrospective falsification

This refers to the unintentional distortion of memory that occurs when it is filtered through a person's current emotional, experiential and cognitive state. It is often found in depressed patients, but any mental illness can lead to retrospective falsification.

23. F Reduced vision following cataract operation

This is seen in cases of old age psychosis or paraphrenia in which the patient is deprived of sensation such as hearing or reduced vision. Secondary to this, they can have experiences such as visual or auditory hallucinations.

24. E History of rape in childhood

There is no convincing evidence of a genetic component in the aetiology of borderline personality. Psychoanalytic theories propose a disturbed relationship with her mother at the stage of the child's individuality. These patients are more likely to report physical and sexual abuse in childhood, although prospective studies have not been reported.

25. D Having been raped 4 months ago

The necessary cause of post-traumatic stress disorder (PTSD) is an exceptionally stressful event. Such an event can involve actual or threatened death or serious injury or a threat to the physical integrity of the person or others. Vulnerability to developing PTSD appears to be related to temperament and in particular neuroticism. Classic conditioning may be involved. The cognitive model of PTSD suggests that, when the normal processing of emotionally charged information is overwhelmed, memories persist in an unprocessed form in which they can intrude into conscious awareness.

26. A Grief reaction

This is the involuntary emotional and behavioural response to bereavement. It is a continuous process but it can be described conveniently as three stages. The first stage lasts from a few hours to several days; the second stage lasts from a few weeks to about 6 months but may be much longer. In the third stage, the symptoms of grief reaction subside and everyday activities are resumed.

27. G Severe depressive episode with psychotic symptoms

The patient presents with symptoms consistent with severe depression with psychotic symptoms. Auditory hallucination, in this case, is mood congruent, although it could be non-congruent. In addition, this condition can present with nihilistic delusions, serious suicidal thoughts and plans.

28. E Diogenes syndrome

This is characterised by hoarding of unnecessary objects and rubbish, gross self-neglect and a refusal to accept help. This condition is usually found in elderly people but not necessarily so. The patients are often intelligent and wealthy. About half of them have no previous psychiatric history, but some have a history of paranoid personality disorder or being socially isolated. On average, half these patients are not mentally ill and the rest have schizophrenia, dementia, depression, obsessive–compulsive disorder or a stress reaction in a certain type of personality.

29. F Fregoli's syndrome

This is a misidentification syndrome characterised by a delusional belief that various people, including strangers whom the person meets, are really the same people but in disguise. They then spy on the patient who believes that he or she is being followed or persecuted by them.

30. G Othello's syndrome

This is also called pathological morbid jealousy. It is a delusional belief or an overvalued idea that leads a person to believe that his or her partner/spouse is unfaithful. It occurs more often in men than in women. It may have no basis and can present on its own. It may be a manifestation of alcohol abuse, cocaine abuse, schizophrenia, paranoid personality disorder and delusional disorder. It may lead to stalking, searching, aggressive demands for proof and violence. Its treatment includes managing the underlying condition and sometimes a permanent separation.

31. G, I Schema of permanent object. Symbolisation

Piaget's theory is concerned with the process by which innate motor reflexes are gradually transformed and develop into mature, psychological structures of adults, capable of abstract thinking and reasoning. It is a stage theory which means that children are seen as passing through a sequence of stages, a predetermined hierarchy, in an invariant order. It is characterised by a lack of object permanence and emergence of symbolic representation.

32. C, H Egocentricity. Semiotic function

Operations are mental sequences of actions that follow a logical pattern. The preoperational child has not developed this logical ability. Piaget considered these children to be egocentric, being unable to consider the world from any viewpoint other than their own.

Semiotic function means that children represent something with a signifier which serves as a representative function, e.g. drawing is used initially as a playful exercise but eventually signifies the real world.

33. B, E, J Conservation. Operational thought. Syncretic reasoning

Children develop the concept of conservation when they realise that the quantity or amount of a substance or group of objects remains unchanged if nothing has been added to or taken away from it. Syncretic reasoning means that the items are classified by a single and changing criterion. Transductive reasoning means that inferences are made about relationships based on a single attribute. This influences the development of animistic thinking, i.e. the inanimate objects are seen as being alive.

34. F Reversibility

It is the capacity to understand that one thing can turn into another and back again, e.g. water and ice.

35. G Combination of permissive and loving

These parents treat their children as equal.

36. C Combination of authoritarian and hostile

These parents make unrealistic demands and punish the child to control his or her behaviour.

37. J Permissive

These parents make few demands and also provide less guidance and support.

38. D Combination of authoritarian and loving

These parents try to balance their authority, love and affection.

There are different types of parenting skills. They are mainly divided into the basis of warmth and level of control displayed by parents on a regular basis in various situations.

39. D Millon clinical multiaxial inventory

This provides an individual profile, an interpretative report and a categorical assessment of personality limited to borderline, schizotypal and paranoid types.

40. F The Personality assessment schedule

This generates diagnosis for both the ICD-10 and the DSM-IV. The emphasis is on the premorbid personality traits. It takes about 30–40 minutes to administer.

41. E Neuroticism, extroversion, openness, personality inventory

This is easy for participants to use. It has a disadvantage of being incapable of distinguishing mental state features from personality traits.

42. J Structured clinical interview for the DSM-IV personality

This assesses the DSM-IV and ICD-10 personality disorders either categorically or dimensionally. It is a semi-structured clinical interview with 101 questions in a thematic version and 107 questions in a disorder-by-disorder version.

43. C International personality disorders examination

This assesses both the DSM-IV and ICD-10 personality disorders categorically and/or dimensionally. It is a semi-structured clinical interview in the DSM-IV (99 sets of questions) and the ICD-10 (67 sets of questions) versions.

44. F Tangentiality

This is a form of thought disorder. It applies to answering questions in a manner in which the answer is partially relevant or completely irrelevant.

45. E Perseveration

This is a form of thought disorder in which the patient is unable to shift from tasks or activity. It is an abnormal response to a stimulus, resulting in repetition of words or phrases even after the stimulus has ceased.

46. A Circumstantiality

This occurs when a person's thinking proceeds slowly with many unnecessary and trivial details, and finally it reaches the point. The goal of thinking is never completely lost but thinking proceeds towards it by an intricate and convoluted path.

47. J Semantic memory

This is also called a fact memory which is responsible for long-term storage of various things.

Retrospective falsification means the unintentional distortion of memory which occurs when it is filtered through a person's current emotional, experiential and cognitive state.

48. A Confabulation

This is the falsification of memory occurring in clear consciousness in association with organic pathology.

49. E, G, H Recognition. Registration. Retrieval

Short-term store (STS) and long-term store (LTS) are linked so that information in STS may be transferred into LTS for long-term storage.

50. D Jamais-vu

This is the knowledge that an event has been experienced before but is not currently associated with the appropriate feeling of familiarity.

51. F This operates on the principle of pleasure. It is unable to delay gratification and needs immediate pleasure of its instinctual urges. It engages in primary process thinking, which is fantasy oriented and operates at the unconscious level.

52. G This operates according to the reality principle, delays the gratification, engages in secondary process thinking which is oriented towards problem solving and operates at all three levels of awareness.

53. B Moral component of personality, emerges at 3–5 years of age, and operates at all three levels of awareness

According to Freud:

Id: primitive and instinctive component, operates on pleasure principle
Ego: decision-making component, operates on reality principle
Super-ego: moral component

54. D 6–12 years of age

See **Table 4.1** for further information.

55. B 2–3 years of age

See **Table 4.1** for further information.

56. C 4–5 years of age

See **Table 4.1** for further information.

57. E Puberty onwards

See **Table 4.1** for further information.

58. A 0–1 year of age

See **Table 4.1** for further information.

Table 4.1 Freud's stages of psychosexual development			
Freud's stages of psychosexual development			
Stage	Approximate ages	Erotic focus	Key tasks and experiences
Oral	0–1 years	Mouth (sucking, biting)	Weaning (from breast or bottle); fixation could form the basis of obsessive eating or smoking later in life
Anal	2–3 years	Anus (expelling or retaining faeces)	Toilet training; fixation could form the basis of obsessions and compulsions later on
Phallic	4–5 years	Genitals (masturbating)	Identifying with adult role models; coping with oedipal crisis and penis envy
Latency	6–2 years	None (sexually repressed)	Expanding social contacts
Genital	Puberty onwards	Genitals (being sexually intimate)	Establishing intimate relationships; contributing to society through working

59. A Amok

This is the culture-bond condition that is originally from Malaysia. It is a dissociative state characterised by a period of brooding, which is followed by anger or violent outburst. It can lead to homicidal behaviour, and is found only in men. A person returns to his premorbid state after sometime.

60. C Dhat

This is the term used in India. It is the state of severe anxiety and hypochondriacal belief that semen is discharged into the urine. The person feels lethargic, weak and exhausted.

61. H Piblokoto

This is the dissociative episode which consists of an extreme form of excitement. It can last up to 30 minutes and is followed by convulsive state or coma, which can last up to 12 hours. It is found in Eskimo communities. During the attack, a person can tear off his or her clothes, break things or eat faeces.

62. G Pa-leng

This is the culture-bond syndrome that is seen in China. Here the person has excessive fear of cold and wears lots of clothing to prevent it.

63. D Ganser's syndrome

Approximate answers suggest that the patient understands the questions but appears to be deliberately avoiding the correct answer. Ganser's syndrome was believed to be a hysterical condition with unconscious production of symptoms to avoid a court appearance. Many now believe that it is indicative of either an organic or a psychotic state rather than a hysterical one as originally believed.

64. F Klüver–Bucy syndrome

This occurs when both right and left medial temporal lobes of the brain malfunction. The patient explores objects by putting them in the mouth. He or she engages in inappropriate sexual behaviour, and presents with visual agnosia, loss of normal fear, anger responses, memory loss, distractibility, seizures and dementia. It may be associated with herpes encephalitis and trauma. Treatment is symptomatic and supportive. It is not life threatening. The amygdala has been particularly implicated in the pathogenesis of this syndrome.

65. H Ramsay Hunt syndrome

Ramsay Hunt syndrome is due to reactivation of the varicella-zoster virus in the geniculate ganglion of the facial nerve. In this syndrome, a red painful rash is associated with blisters in the ears or mouth, and unilateral facial paralysis, ear pain, hearing loss, dizziness, dry eye and changes in taste sensations. A polymerase chain reaction on fluid from blisters demonstrates viral genetic material.

66. E Gilles de la Tourette's syndrome

This is an idiopathic condition in which multiple tics are associated with forced involuntary vocalisations, which may take the form of obscenities (coprolalia). It is characterised by a combination of multiple motor and vocal tics that wax and wane. Other features include echolalia, coprophagia, concerns with symmetry, aggressive thoughts, forced touching, fear of self-harm, fear of cleanliness and hygiene. Depressive symptoms are common and attention deficit hyperactivity disorder has been described.

67. C Emotional disorder with onset specific to childhood

In this scenario, the girl is 5 years old and has a persistent fear of strangers. Her symptoms are consistent with a diagnosis of emotional disorder with onset specific to childhood, precisely social anxiety disorder of childhood. It should be noted that some degree of anxiety, fear and apprehension towards strangers and new situations is present in childhood. However, in social anxiety disorder of childhood, the symptoms begin before the age of 6 years and are persistent.

68. K Tic disorder

The most common form of tic disorder in children is transient tic disorder. It can be in the form of eye blinking, facial grimacing or head jerking. It is frequently seen in a child around age 5 years and usually disappears within 12 months of the onset.

69. D Hyperkinetic disorder

This case scenario is suggestive of hyperkinetic disorder. It is characterised by impulsivity, hyperactivity and inattention. For diagnosis, it should be present before the age of 7 years and symptoms should be present in at least two different environments, e.g. at school and at home.

70. E Mixed disorder of conduct and emotions

The case scenario is consistent with mixed disorder of conduct and emotions. As the name suggests, there is evidence of a conduct disorder such as antisocial, defiant and aggressive behaviour. The patient may also present with emotional symptoms of affect and mood such as anxiety and depression.

71. C Emotional disorder with onset specific to childhood

This case scenario is consistent with an emotional disorder with onset specific to childhood, specifically phobic anxiety disorder of childhood. This disorder can include a wide range of objects and situations. In the scenario, the girl has an excessive fear of crowded places and refuses to go shopping although has no problem going to the local shop.

Chapter 5

Mock examination

Questions: EMIs

Theme: Formal thought disorder

Options for questions: 1–3

A   Circumstantiality
B   Clang association
C   Drivelling
D   Flight of ideas

E   Neologism
F   Omission
G   Tangentiality

For each of the following cases, select the single most appropriate thought disorder. Each option may be used once, more than once or not at all.

1.   A 32-year-old patient with mania spoke rapidly with pressure of speech and jumped from one topic to another.

2.   A 40-year-old patient with schizophrenia used new words or phrases in place of conventional words while speaking.

3.   A 30-year-old patient with schizophrenia gave an answer that was appropriate to the general topic without answering the question.

Theme: Interview techniques

Options for questions: 4–7

A   Clarification
B   Confrontation
C   Direct question
D   Facilitation
E   Leading statement

F   Open question
G   Polythematic question
H   Recapitulation
I   Reflection
J   Silence

For each of the following cases, select the single most appropriate interview technique. Each option may be used once, more than once or not at all.

4.   The interviewer noded his head and said 'Uh-huh, go on …'.

5.   The interviewer begain the assessment with the following: 'How have things been?'

6.   The interviewer refrained from commenting and allowed the patient to cry for a few minutes.

7.   The interviewer felt that there was something that the patient was missing or denying and stated: 'What you have done might have killed you. You said you wanted to end your life but you immediately called the ambulance and sent a text to your mother. It seemed that you were feeling stuck and wanted some help.'

Theme: Applications of memory tests

Options for questions: 8–10

A   Benton's visual retention test
B   California verbal learning test
C   Objective learning test
D   Paired associate learning test

E   Rey–Osterrieth complex figure test
F   Rivermead behavioural memory test
G   Synonym learning test

For each of the following description of a test, select the single most appropriate memory test. Each option may be used once, more than once or not at all.

8.   This is a memory test devised by Wilson which lays emphasis on daily living skills. Its subtests include orientation, name recall, route memory and picture recognition.

9.   This is a visual memory test where the patient is presented with a complex design.

10. This is a visual recall test where designs are presented to the patient for 10 seconds, after which he or she attempts to recall and draw the design. It can be used to exclude visuoperceptual problems.

Theme: Mini-mental state examination

Options for questions: 11–13

A   Comprehension
B   Concentration
C   Construction
D   Delayed recall

E   Long-term recall
F   Naming
G   Orientation to time
H   Writing

For each of the items of the MMSE, select the single most likely cognitive process that is being tested. Each option may be used once, more than once or not at all.

11. Asking for current season

12. Copying 'interlocking hexagons'

13. Serial sevens test

Theme: Diagnosis of movement disorders

Options for questions: 14–16

A   Akathisia
B   Athetosis
C   Cataplexy
D   Dystonic reaction

E   Hemiballismus
F   Myoclonus
G   Spasmodic torticollis

For each of the following cases, select the single most correct sign that describes it best. Each option may be used once, more than once or not at all.

14. A 40-year-old man experienced brief sudden loss of muscle power, leading to falls when he laughed. He remained fully awake during these attacks.

15. A 42-year-old man involuntarily pulled his head towards his right side and twisted his face towards the left side for a few minutes. He sometimes held his chin with his hand to prevent these uncomfortable movements.

16. A 21-year-old man developed persistent feelings to move 1 hour after being started on an antipsychotic drug.

Theme: Assessment of withdrawal syndromes

Options for questions: 17–19

A	Alcohol	E	Diazepam
B	Amitriptyline	F	Heroin
C	Cannabis	G	Paroxetine
D	Cocaine	H	Tobacco

For each of the following set of withdrawal symptoms, select the single most likely drug involved. Each option may be used once, more than once or not at all.

17. Tremors of hands, churning in stomach, nausea and sweating

18. Rhinorrhoea, piloerection, yawning, papillary dilatation

19. Dysphoric mood, increased appetite, fatigue

Theme: Assessment of memory deficits

Options for questions: 20–24

A	Anterograde memory impairment	F	Jamais-vu
B	Confabulation	G	Pseudologia fantastica
C	Déjà-vu	H	Reduplicative paramnesia
D	Delusional misinterpretation of memory	I	Retrograde amnesia
E	Implicit memory impairment	J	Semantic memory impairment

For each of the following cases, select the single most likely memory deficit or psychopathology. Each option may be used once, more than once or not at all.

20. A 53-year-old man with a long history of alcohol abuse was noted to invent details for events that he couldn't remember.

21. A 39-year-old Catholic woman was walking down an alley in Mumbai and felt that she had been there before when in fact this was her first visit to India.

22. A 30-year-old woman believed that after a breast operation her soul had been removed from her body.

23. A 55-year-old businessman believed that he had two identical houses, one in London and the other in New York.

24. A 58-year-old man did not remember what road he was driving on after a road traffic accident.

Theme: ICD-10 diagnosis of psychotic disorders

Options for questions: 25–27

A Catatonic behaviour such as posturing or excitement
B Flattening of affect and loss of volition
C Disorganised thoughts and incoherent speech

D Onset in adolescents or young adults
E Onset in later life
F Prominent delusions and/or hallucinations
G Schizoid personality

For each of the following cases, select the most appropriate feature(s). Each option may be used once, more than once or not at all.

25. Paranoid schizophrenia (select ONE option)

26. Hebephrenic schizophrenia (select THREE options)

27. Persistent delusional disorder (select TWO options)

Theme: Diagnosis of personality disorders

Options for questions: 28–31

A Anankastic personality disorder
B Anxious personality disorder
C Dissocial personality disorder
D Emotionally unstable personality disorder – borderline type
E Emotionally unstable personality disorder – impulsive type

F Histrionic personality disorder
G Paranoid personality disorder
H Narcissistic personality disorder
I Schizoid personality disorder
J Schizotypal personality disorder

For each of the following cases, select the single most likely diagnosis. Each option may be used once, more than once or not at all.

28. A 35-year-old man was excessively sensitive to setbacks and had a tendency to bear grudges.

29. A 30-year-old man displayed emotional coldness, preferred solitary activities and had no desire for close and confiding relationships.

30. A 40-year-old man was not concerned about the feelings of others and persistently disregarded social norms.

31. A 23-year-old woman had tendencies to get involved in intense and unstable relationships, avoid abandonment and chronic feelings of emptiness.

Theme: Kohlberg's moral development

Options for questions: 32–35

A Level 1: preconventional morality
B Level 2: preconventional morality
C Level 3: conventional morality

D Level 4: conventional morality
E Level 5: postconventional morality
F Level 6: postconventional morality

For each of the following descriptions, select the single most likely stage of moral development. Each option may be used once, more than once or not at all.

32. Good boy/good girl orientation: 'I won't do it because I want people to like me.'

33. Obeying rules to avoid punishments.

34. Maintains social rules and laws: 'I won't do it because it would break the law.'

35. 'I won't do it because I am not obliged to do it.'

Theme: Clinical applications of neuropsychological tests

Options for questions: 36–42

A   Test of abstract thinking

B   Test of conceptualisation

C   Test of constructional abilities

D   Test of intelligence

E   Test of judgement

F   Test of motor sequencing

G   Test of premorbid IQ

H   Test of pure attention

I   Test of response inhibition

J   Test of set shifting

K   Test of verbal memory

L   Test of visual memory

For each of the following tests, select the single most appropriate use. Each option may be used once, more than once or not at all.

36. Cognitive estimates test

37. Go–no-go test

38. Luria three-step test

39. National adult reading test

40. Proverb interpretation

41. Raven's progressive matrices

42. Wisconsin card sorting test

theme: Disorders of perception

Options for questions: 43–46

A   Affect illusion

B   Complete illusion

C   Dysmegalopsia

D   Hypnagogic hallucination

E   Hypnopompic hallucination

F   Kinaesthetic hallucination

G   Pareidolia

H   Phantom mirror image

I   Visual hyperaesthesia

For each of the following descriptions, select the single most likely psychopathology that best describes it. Each option may be used once, more than once or not at all.

43. It is a visual experience in which individuals see an image of themselves in external space viewed from within their own body.

44. This refers to a change in the perceived shape of an object.

45. This refers to misreading words in newspapers or misreading misprints because we read words as if they were complete.

46. This refers to increased intensity of sensations which may be the result of intense emotions or lowering of the physiological threshold.

Theme: Object relations theory

Options for questions: 47–49

A	Depressive anxiety	G	Persecutory depressive anxiety
B	Depressive position	H	Persecutory schizoid position
C	Paranoid anxiety	I	Projective identification
D	Paranoid schizoid position	J	Schizoid anxiety
E	Paranoid schizotypal position	K	Splitting
F	Persecutory anxiety		

For each of the following descriptions, select the most appropriate concept from the list above. Each option may be used once, more than once or not at all.

47. Mother is viewed ambivalently as having both positive and negative aspects, and as the target for a mixture of loving and hateful feelings.

48. An infant projects derivatives of the death instinct onto the mother and then fears attack from the 'bad mother'.

49. This is an infant's mode of organising experience in which all aspects of infant and mother are split into good and bad elements.

Theme: Psychodynamic concepts

Options for questions: 50–54

A	Adolph Meyer	G	Erik Erikson
B	Alfred Adler	H	Heinz Kohut
C	Carl Jung	I	Karen Horney
D	Carl Rogers	J	Melanie Klein
E	Donald Winnicott	K	Otto Kernberg
F	Eric Berne	L	Otto Rank

For each of the following concepts and theories stages, select the name of the person from the list above who proposed that. Each option may be used once, more than once or not at all.

50. All persons have three ego states that exist within them: the child, the adult and the parent.

51. A child's sibling position (birth order in the family of origin) results in life-long influences on character and lifestyle.

52. Anima refers to a man's undeveloped femininity whereas animus refers to a woman's undeveloped masculinity.

53. This is the concept of narcissism and self-psychology.

54. An object, such as a blanket, provides a soothing sense of security in the absence of the mother.

Theme: Clinical applications of ego defence mechanisms

Options for questions: 55–57

A   Altruism
B   Displacement
C   Isolation
D   Projection

E   Regression
F   Repression
G   Splitting
H   Undoing

For each of the following cases, select the single most likely defence mechanism used. Each option may be used once, more than once or not at all.

55.   A 33-year-old married woman was unaware of her hatred towards her father. However, she often felt inexplicably resentful towards older men in positions of authority. She could not understand why she had felt like this for a long time.

56.   A 30-year-old single man adored his mother but was cold, distant and resentful towards his father most of his life. He was unaware of his hidden sexual interest in his mother and his death wish for his father.

57.   A 64-year-old man thought 'his 82-year-old mother will fall ill and die'. He regarded such a thought as an alien, intensive idea that had no real connection with him. It did not arouse guilt or feelings of wishfulness.

Theme: Concepts in cultural psychiatry

Options for questions: 58–59

A   Anthropology
B   Culture
C   Cultural identity
D   Prejudice

E   Ethnicity
F   Race
G   Religion
H   Stigma

For each of the following descriptions, select the single most likely concept from above. Each option may be used once, more than once or not at all.

58.   It refers to meanings, values and behavioural norms that are learned and transmitted with in the society and its social groups.

59.   It consists of groups of individuals sharing a common ancestry, shared beliefs, history, special rites of passage, rituals and family roles.

Theme: Diagnosis of dementia

Options for question: 60–63

A   Alzheimer's dementia
B   Frontotemporal dementia
C   Lewy body dementia
D   Normal pressure hydrocephalus

E   Pick's disease
F   Progressive supranuclear palsy
G   Semantic dementia
H   Vascular dementia

For each of the following case, select the single most likely diagnosis. Each option may be used once, more than once or not at all.

60.   This is the commonest form of dementia in developed countries.

61.   Pathological findings include ballooned neurons and 'knife-blade' atrophy of the frontal and temporal poles.

62.   This is early onset dementia with features including *Witzelsucht* and apathy.

63.   This involves dilated ventricles with progressive memory loss and urinary incontinence.

Theme: Disorders of sexual preference and gender identity disorders

Options for questions: 64–66

A Individual dressing in clothing of the opposite sex in order to be a member of that gender
B Closely associated with sexual arousal, the person removes clothes after orgasm
C Minimum period of 3 months required
D Minimum period of 6 months required
E No intention to have sexual intercourse with the person observed
F Persistent or recurrent urge to watch people engaging in sexual or intimate behaviour
G Individual dressing in clothing of the opposite sex to have temporary membership of that gender
H Preference for sexual activity, as a recipient or provider, involving bondage
I No sexual motivation for the cross-dressing
J Recurrent or persistent desire to expose the genitalia to strangers

For each of the following gender identity disorders, select the options from above as instructed. Each option may be used once, more than once or not at all.

64. Fetishistic transvestism (select **THREE** options).

65. Voyeurism (select **THREE** options).

66. Sadomasochism (select **TWO** options).

Theme: Diagnosis of neurotic disorders

Options for questions: 67–70

A Body dysmorphic disorder
B Generalised anxiety disorder
C Hypochondriacal disorder
D Obsessive–compulsive disorder
E Panic disorder
F Post-traumatic stress disorder
G Somatisation disorder
H Specific phobia

For each of the following descriptions, select the most likely diagnosis as instructed. Each option may be used once, more than once or not at all.

67. These are included in the subcategories of other anxiety disorders (select TWO options).

68. There are repetitive thoughts for 2 weeks, followed by ritualistic behaviours (select ONE option).

69. There is a history of 2 years of symptoms. There is a preoccupation with complaints of physical symptoms (select ONE option).

70. There is a preoccupation with at least two serious physical diseases for a minimum period of 6 months. There is a persistent refusal to accept medical reassurance (select ONE option).

Theme: Differential diagnosis of dementia

Options for questions: 71–73

A	Alzheimer's dementia	E	Lewy body dementia
B	Down's syndrome	F	Multi-infarct dementia
C	Frontotemporal dementia	G	Normal pressure hydrocephalus
D	Huntington's disease	H	Vascular dementia

For each of the following cases, select the single most likely diagnosis. Each option may be used once, more than once or not at all.

71. A 64-year-old man presented with a 2-year history of memory problems. Recently, there has been deterioration in speech and the ability to dress himself.

72. A 54-year-old man presented with inappropriate social behaviour, disinhibition, increased talkativeness and reckless behaviour. His MMSE score was 25/30.

73. A 59-year-old man presented with difficulty walking, memory problems and difficulty controlling his bladder.

Theme: Mechanism of action of psychotropic drugs

Options for questions: 74–78

A	5-HT$_{1A}$ Receptor agonist	F	Long-acting opioid agonist
B	α_2-Receptor agonist	G	Monoamine oxidase B (MAO-B) inhibitor
C	D$_2$-Receptor antagonist	H	Partial opioid agonist
D	D$_2$-Receptor partial agonist	I	Reversible MAO-A inhibitor
E	Long-acting μ-antagonist	J	Short-acting μ-antagonist

For each of the following drugs, select the single most likely mechanism of action. Each option may be used once, more than once or not at all.

74. Aripiprazole

75. Selegiline

76. Buspirone

77. Buprenorphine

78. Naltrexone

Answers: EMIs

1. D Flight of ideas

These can be found when analysing the speech of a patient with mania or hypomania. Here the thought moves abruptly from idea to idea and is often expressed through rapid and pressured speech.

2. E Neologism

This is seen in patients with schizophrenia when the patient invents new words or phrases in an idiosyncratic way.

3. G Tangentiality

This is a situation in which the individual's response to a question is with a reply that is appropriate to the general topic without answering the main question.

Word salad, circumstantiality, clang association, drivelling, omissions, flight of ideas, neologism and tangentiality all are types of formal thought disorders.

4. D Facilitation

This is used to show acknowledgement and allow the interview to progress.

5. F Open question

Open/broad questions open up an interview and allow a free exchange of information.

6. J Silence

This can allow time for the patient to digest, accept or contemplate.

7. B Confrontation

This is used when the interviewer suspects that the patient may be missing or denying something.

The following are techniques used in clinical interviews:

- Clarification: to check the interviewer's understanding and gather further information.
- Direct question: these are targeted at uncovering specific information about a certain topic.
- Leading statement: can influence the interviewee's responses.
- Polythematic question: exploring more than one area at a time.
- Recapitulation: process of summarising.
- Reflection: a supportive way of repeating, although not exactly, what the patient has said.

8. F Rivermead behavioural memory test

This is used for testing daily memory problems. It is also helpful to test whether there is any change over a period of time and other abilities. Some of the subset includes a orientation, name recall, route memory and picture recognition.

9. E Rey–Osterrieth complex figure test

The Rey–Osterrieth complex figure test involves asking the patient to copy a complex figure that is shown to him or her, then both the figure and the copy are removed and the patient is asked to draw it again.

10. A Benton's visual retention test

Benton visual retention test examines the ability to copy and recall a variety of figures and tests.

The California verbal learning test measures verbal learning and variety of memory including retention and retrieval.

11. G Orientation to time

The MMSE is a screening tool for dementia. It tests various cognitive functions as follows.

Orientation to time and place gives 5 points each. One of them asks for the current season.

12. C Construction

Constructional ability is tested by asking the patient to copy a diagram of interlocking pentagons.

13. B Concentration

The serial sevens tests and spelling 'world' backwards are used to assess attention and calculation.

14. C Cataplexy

Cataplexy (sudden bilateral loss of muscle tone triggered by a strong emotional reaction) is one of the four classic symptoms of narcolepsy. Narcolepsy is the commonest neurological cause of hypersomnia and affects men and women equally. Excessive sleepiness, sleep paralysis and hypnagogic hallucinations are the other three symptoms of narcoplepsy.

15. G Spasmodic torticollis

In spasmodic torticollis, there is a spasm of the neck muscles, especially sternomastoid, which pulls the head towards the same side and twists the face in the opposite direction. At first, the spasm lasts for a few minutes but it gradually increases until the neck is permanently twisted.

16. A Akathisia

This is an unpleasant inner restlessness and an urge to move, either individual body parts or the whole body (e.g. pacing up and down). It occurs in up to 40% of patients within 2 weeks of receiving first-generation antipsychotic drugs. Incidence rates with newer drugs are unclear but seem to be lower.

17. A Alcohol

It is important to remember that concomitant infection, Wernicke's encephalopathy, metabolic disturbance, hypoglycaemia and head injury may complicate the clinical picture and prognosis.

18. F Heroin

The opiate-withdrawal syndrome is characterised by nausea, vomiting, muscle aches, lacrimation, sweating, diarrhoea, fever and insomnia, in addition to other given symptoms and signs.

19. D Cocaine

The 'crash' typically occurs within 30 minutes and may last up to 40 hours. The withdrawal phase tends to peak at 2–4 days and various depressive symptoms last for several weeks after that. There is no specific symptomatic treatment.

20. B Confabulation

This is the falsification of memory occurring in clear consciousness, in association with organic brain pathology. It diminishes as the impairment worsens.

21. C Déjà-vu

This is not strictly a disturbance of memory, but a problem with the familiarity of places and events. It comprises the feeling of having experienced a current event in the past, even though it has no basis.

22. D Delusional misinterpretation of memory

Delusional memories are variously defined. The present state examination suggests that they are experiences of past events that did not occur but which the patient clearly 'remembers'. They have two components: the perception (real or imagined) and the memory.

23. H Reduplicative paramnesia

This is the delusion that a double of a person or place exists elsewhere. The phenomenon suggests non-dominant parietal lobe pathology and is related to other disturbances of recognition. It is also called doppelganger.

24. I Retrograde amnesia

This is the inability to recall previously learned material. However, memories from the remote past remain intact, as does recall of over-learned material from the past and immediate recall.

25. F Prominent delusions and/or hallucinations

Patients with paranoid schizophrenia usually present with a delusional belief of a paranoid nature. In addition, they can present with hallucinations, predominantly auditory in nature.

26. B, C, D Flattening of affect and loss of volition. Disorganised thoughts and incoherent speech. Onset in adolescents or young adults

Symptoms of hebephrenic schizophrenia usually present in adolescents or young adults. Patients have flat affect and loss of volition. Their speech is incoherent and thoughts may appear to be disorganised. In this subtype of schizophrenia, delusions and hallucinations are not prominent and if present are fleeting in nature and not well formed.

27. E, F Onset in later life; prominent delusions and/or hallucinations

In persistent delusional disorder, the onset is usually in later life. Patients present with an encapsulated delusional belief and this may be the only symptom present.

28. G Paranoid personality disorder

Personality disorders are a severe disturbance in one's personality and behavioural tendencies, which have not directly resulted from disease or damage to the brain. They are associated with significant distress at the personal and social level. They are usually manifested in childhood and continue throughout adolescence. Paranoid personality disorder is characterised by excessive sensitivity to setbacks, suspiciousness, unforgiveness and a tendency to misinterpret the action of others as hostile, and recurrent suspiciousness about the sexual fidelity of the spouse/partner.

29. I Schizoid personality disorder

This is characterised by withdrawal from close, confiding relationships and other social contacts. There is a preference for fantasy and solitary activities. There is also a limited capacity to express feelings and experience pleasure.

30. C Dissocial personality disorder

This is characterised by disregard for social norms and obligations. There is callous unconcern for the feelings of others. Behaviour is not modified, even after punishment. There is low tolerance to frustration and a low threshold to discharge aggression. There is also a tendency to blame others.

31. D Emotionally unstable personality disorder – borderline type

This is characterised by a tendency to act impulsively without considering the consequences. Mood is unpredictable and there is a tendency for emotional outburst. It can be the impulsive or borderline type. The impulsive type is characterised by a marked tendency to act unexpectedly, quarrelsome behaviour, outbusts of anger and violence, difficulty in maintaining any course of action and unpredictable mood. The borderline type is characterised by uncertainty or disturbance in self-image, a tendency to get involved in intense and unstable relationships, excessive efforts to avoid abandonment, recurrent threats or acts of self-harm, and chronic feelings of emptiness.

32. C Level 3: conventional morality

The study of moral development has been dominated by Kohlberg's moral stages divided into three levels and six stages. According to Kohlberg, at birth all humans have no moral or ethical stance. People proceed through these stages in the same order. The three levels are:

1. Preconventional (7–12 years to middle childhood)
2. Conventional (13–16 years)
3. Postconventional (16–20 years).

Very few people reach stage 6 and the most advanced stage, in which the patients' view is based on abstract principles, cross-cultural studies have confirmed the universal applicability of these stages. Social norms are seen as the mainstay of ethical behaviour. Social order is taken into account at the expense of immediate concrete outcomes, which is typical of young teenagers. This is a stage of good interpersonal relationships. Children can see their own actions from the perspective of another person.

33. A Level 1: preconventional morality

Morality is externally governed by the consequences of an action. Actions that are punished are seen as bad because they are punished. Children conform to the rules imposed on them by adults, who are more powerful than they are. This is a stage of obedience and punishment orientation. Avoidance of punishment is the key factor in the child's understanding of right and wrong.

34. D Level 4: conventional morality

This is a stage of maintaining the social order. The child now expands the idea of fair behaviour or just motives, and sees laws and judgements as those that are applied equally to all members of society. The morality of an action is defined with reference to society as a whole and in particular conforming to laws. These laws are seen as preventing chaos and being fair for all members of society. Moral behaviour obeys these laws.

35. E Level 5: postconventional morality

This is a stage of social contract and individual rights. Rules are seen as judgements produced by a particular society and the person is aware that alternative rules can be developed that will produce a different type of society. There is a balance between moral justice and the upholding of generally workable laws.

36. B Test of conceptualisation

Cognitive estimates test helps to find how much a person can conceptualise. The person is asked to answer questions that usually don't have accurate answers, e.g. 'How many elephants are in England'. The person is supposed to guess and answer. It is a frontal lobe test.

37. I Test of response inhibition

Go–no-go test is again a test for frontal lobe function. The patient is asked to place a hand on the table and raise one finger in response to single tap. If there are two taps then the patient, should keep still. This is a test to assess response inhibition.

38. F Test of motor sequencing

The Luria's motor sequencing test helps to find how a person follows motor sequences. It is a three-stage test. A person with frontal lobe damage will come out with difficulty moving from one act to the next (fist, palm and side).

39. G Test of premorbid IQ

The national adult reading test assesses the premorbid IQ of an individual.

40. A Test of abstract thinking

Abstract thinking is tested using two tests: proverb interpretation and similarities test. In the test, a person is asked to describe the similarity between two objects. It is a frontal lobe test.

41. D Test of intelligence

Raven's progressive matrices are useful to assess the IQ of an individual who can't read or write English.

42. J Test of set shifting

The Wisconsin card sorting test (WCST) is a test of frontal lobe function. A person has to carry out a set-shifting task in the WCST. Perseverative errors are common.

43. H Phantom mirror image

This is also known as autoscopy. It is not just a visual hallucination, because kinaesthetic and somatic sensation must also be present to give the patient the impression that the hallucination is oneself.

44. C Dysmegatopsia

This refers to a change in the perceived shape of an object. It could be micropsia, in which the patients sees an object as smaller than it really is, or macropsia, which is an opposite kind of visual experience. It can result from retinal disease, disorders of accommodation and convergence, and temporal and parietal lobe lesions.

45. B Complete illusion

This depends on inattention, such as misreading in newspapers or missing misprints.

46. I Visual hyperaesthesia

Anxiety and depressive disorders, as well as hangovers from alcohol and migraine, are associated with increased sensitivity to noise.

47. B Depressive position

When children internalise a secure good-enough view of themselves, they would move from a paranoid–schizoid position to the depressive position, in which the mother is viewed ambivalently as having both positive and negative aspects and as the target of a mixture of loving and hateful feelings. These two positions are never fully resolved and adult life is a mixture of functioning in both of these. This results in a reversion to the paranoid–schizoid position under stress, and returning to the reality-oriented depressive position when more secure and supported.

48. F Persecutory anxiety

Melanie Klein evolved a theory of internal object relations. She viewed projection and introjection as the primary defensive operations in the first months of life. Infants project derivatives of the death instinct into the mother and then fear attack from the 'bad mother'. This is referred to as persecutory anxiety.

49. D Paranoid schizoid position

According to Melanie Klein, infants have anxiety that is caused by the death instinct which is developed due to birth trauma, hunger and frustration. The infant splits the mother and other objects into good and bad component. According to Klein this splitting is important for normal development of infants.

50. F Eric Berne

Berne developed the concept of transactional analysis. Transaction is a stimulus presented by one person which evokes a corresponding response in another. He also defined psychological games and strokes. According to him, all people have three ego states that exist within them: the child, the adult and the parent (see **Table 5.1**).

51. B Alfred Adler

Adler introduced the term 'masculine protest' to describe the tendency to move from a passive, feminine role to an active, masculine role. He described an inferiority complex and organ inferiority. He suggested that the firstborn child reacts with anger to the birth of siblings and struggles against giving up the powerful position of being the only child (see **Table 5.1**).

52. C Carl Jung

Jung's school of psychology is known as analytical psychology. He expanded Freud's concept of the unconscious by describing the collective unconscious, which includes archetypes. He noted that there are two types of personality organisations: introversion and extraversion. He also described anima (a man's undeveloped femininity) and animus (a woman's undeveloped masculinity) – the unconscious traits possessed by men and women respectively (see **Table 5.1**).

53. H Heinz Kohut

Kohut is best known for his writings on narcissism and the development of self-psychology. He viewed the development and maintenance of self-esteem and self-cohesion as more important than sexuality or aggression (see **Table 5.1**).

54. E Donald Winnicott

Winnicott developed the notion of the transitional object, which serves as a substitute for the mother during an infant's efforts to separate and become independent.

It provides a soothing sense of security in the mother's absence. Ordinarily it is like a pacifier, a blanket or a teddy bear (see **Table 5.1**).

Persons	Concept	Comments
Table 5.1 Eight stages of the life cycle		
1. Adolph Meyer	Theory of psychobiology	Coined the term 'common-sense psychiatry'
2. Alfred Adler	Individual psychology	Inferiority complex, organ inferiority, birth order
3. Carl Jung	Analytical psychology	Personal and collective unconscious, animus and anima, archetypes
4. Carl Rogers	Client-centred theory	Self-actualisation, self-direction
5. Donald Winnicott	Transitional object, good-enough mother	One of the central figures in object relations theory
6. Eric Berne	Transactional analysis	Three ego states – child, adult and parent
7. Erik Erikson	Eight stages of life cycle	If successful resolution of a particular stage does not occur, all subsequent stages will have maladjustment
8. Heinz Kohut	Self-psychology	Narcissism
9. Karen Horney	Holistic psychology	Three separate concepts of self – actual self, real self and idealised self
10. Melanie Klein	Internal object relations theory	Infant goes through persecutory anxiety, paranoid schizoid position and depressive position
11. Otto Kernberg	Object relations theory	Proposed borderline personality organisation
12. Otto Rank	Birth trauma theory	The personality is divided into impulses, emotions and will

55. B Displacement

This is the process by which interest and/or emotion is shifted from one object on to another that is less threatening, so that the latter replaces the former.

56. F Repression

This is characterised by the unconscious forgetting of painful ideas or impulses in order to protect the psyche. It overlaps with denial. It is the process of keeping out and ejecting from the consciousness ideas or impulses that are unacceptable to it.

57. C Isolation

This is also known as intellectualisation and is a defence technique for coping with painful affects; the affect is separated from its content, often by treating it objectively rather than experimentally. In a clinical setting, it is most commonly noted when the patient talks about his or her problems in an intellectual, overly abstract manner and has difficulty describing, recalling and experiencing his or her actual feelings.

58. B Culture

Keesing and Strathern (1998) defined culture as systems of shared ideas, concepts, rules and meanings that underlie, and are expressed in, the ways that human beings live. Any given culture requires a shared worldview in order to manage social cohesion. Culture allows the use of a set of rules of any human group and the imparting of these rules to its descendants through the medium of tradition, art, symbols and rituals. Enculturation represents the growing up in any given culture and adoption of its views. Acculturation describes the process of migrants who undergo a transition from their initial culture to the acquisition of the cultural beliefs of a new culture.

59. E Ethnicity

Ethnicity consists of people who have a common ground, beliefs and rituals. Individuals of the same ethnicity can identify with each other, and have a common ancestry, religious beliefs and rites. These common and shared traits can be real or presumed.

60. A Alzheimer's dementia

This is the commonest form of dementia, increasing with advancing age, followed by vascular dementia. Clinical features include amnesia, aphasia, apraxia and agnosias. It typically presents with gradual onset and a progressive decline in cognitive abilities, with a median time of survival from diagnosis of between 5 and 8 years. A rare familial form can present with early onset with an autosomal dominant mode of inheritance.

61. E Pick's disease

Arnold Pick described Pick's disease. It is a type of frontotemporal dementia and is characterised by certain pathological findings, including knife blade atrophy of the frontal and temporal poles, the presence of Pick's cells, also known as ballooned neurons, and Pick's inclusions.

62. B Frontotemporal dementia

Frontotemporal dementias usually present earlier in life and can be characterised by the presence of behavioural changes rather than cognitive changes which may come later. Symptoms can include those that mimic depression and include apathy, withdrawal and amotivation. The symptoms that can mimic manic states include impulsivity, distractibility, talkativeness and impaired judgement.

63. D Normal pressure hydrocephalus

This is another cause for cognitive impairment. It is caused by an increase in intracranial pressure and an abnormal accumulation of cerebrospinal fluid. A triad of symptoms described includes: cognitive impairment, gait disturbance and urinary incontinence. Treatment may involve the use of a shunt.

64. A, B, C Individual dressing in clothing of the opposite sex in order to be a member of that gender. Closely associated with sexual arousal; the person removes clothes after orgasm. Minimum period of 3 months required

Fetishistic transvestism is a sexual preference disorder whereas dual-role transvestism is a gender identity disorder. In the former, there is sexual arousal in cross-dressing and once orgasm is reached there a desire to remove the dress. In the latter, there is a desire for temporary membership of the opposite gender.

65. C, E, F Minimum period of 3 months required. No intention of having sexual intercourse with the person observed. Persistent or recurrent urge to watch people engaging in sexual or intimate behaviour

The disorder of sexual preference also consists of voyeurism and exhibitionism. The sexual preference disorders have a timescale of being present for at least 6 months. There is a persistent or recurrent desire to observe other people engaging in intimate acts but no desire to have intercourse with them.

66. C, H Minimum period of 3 months required. Preference for sexual activity, as a recipient or provider, involving bondage

Sadomasochism is a preference for sexual activity as a provider or recipient. It is associated with pain or humiliation. This activity is a source of sexual gratification for the individuals.

67. B, E Generalised anxiety disorder. Panic disorder

Generalised anxiety disorder, panic disorder, and mixed anxiety and depression are part of a subcategory of other anxiety disorders. It differs from phobic anxiety disorders because the latter manifest in well-defined situations whereas the former is not restricted to any environmental situation.

68. D Obsessive–compulsive disorder

This is characterised by obsessions and compulsion present for a period of 2 weeks. The obsessions can be thoughts, ideas or impulses. The thoughts belong to the person, and are irrational and unpleasant. The person can resist the thoughts and this is followed by compulsion rituals.

69. G Somatisation disorder

Somatisation has a history of 2 years with complaints of multiple physical symptoms. The symptoms can't be explained by any physical disorder. The preoccupation causes distress.

70. C Hypochondriacal disorder

The symptoms of hypochondrical disorder can be subdivided into preoccupation with either two physical diseases or bodily disfigurement. Reassurance does not help.

71. A Alzheimer's dementia

This is the commonest form of dementia, increasing with advancing age, followed by vascular dementia. Clinical features include amnesia, aphasia, apraxia and agnosias. It typically presents with gradual onset and progressive decline in cognitive abilities, with a median time of survival from diagnosis of between 5 and 8 years. A rare familial form can present with early onset in an autosomal dominant mode of inheritance.

72. C Frontotemporal dementia

Frontotemporal dementias usually present earlier in life and can be characterised by the presence of behavioural changes rather than cognitive changes which may come later. Symptoms can include those that mimic depression: apathy, withdrawal and amotivation. The symptoms, which can mimic the manic state, include impulsivity, distractibility, talkativeness and impaired judgement.

73. G Normal pressure hydrocephalus

This is another cause for cognitive impairment. It is caused by an increase in intracranial pressure and an abnormal accumulation of CSF. A triad of symptoms described includes: cognitive impairment, gait disturbance and urinary incontinence. Treatment may involve the use of a shunt.

74. D D_2-receptor partial agonist

Aripiprazole is a partial D_2-receptor agonist and 5-HT_{2A}-receptor antagonist.

75. G Monoamine oxidase B (MAO-B) inhibitor

Selegiline is a selective MAO-B inhibitor.

76. A 5-HT_{1A}-receptor agonist

Buspirone is a partial 5-HT_{1A}-receptor agonist.

77. H Partial opioid antagonist

Buprenorphine is a partial opiod antagonist.

78. E Long-acting μ-antagonist

Naltrexone is a long-acting μ-antagonist.

Methadone is an opioid receptor antagonist.

Moclobemide is a reversible MAO-A inhibitor.

Buproprion is a dopamine reuptake inhibitor and a noradrenaline reuptake inhibitor

Section 2

MRCPsych Paper 2 EMIs

Chapter 6

Test questions: 1

Questions: EMIs

NEUROSCIENCES: NEUROANATOMY

Theme: Functional neuroanatomy

Options for questions: 1–3

A	Acquired sociopathy	E	Anomia
B	Akinetic mutism	F	Dysprosody
C	Amnesia	G	Motor aphasia
D	Amusia	H	Prosopagnosia

For each of the following areas of localisation, select the single most appropriate symptom or sign. Each option may be used once, more than once or not at all.

1. Basal forebrain

2. Orbital cortex

3. Right side areas 44 and 45 (non-dominant)

NEUROSCIENCES: NEUROENDOCRINOLOGY

Theme: Endocrine tests and their clinical use

Options for questions: 4–7

A	Dexamethasone suppression test	F	Plasma aldosterone and renin measurement
B	Fasting plasma glucose	G	Parathyroid hormone
C	24-hour urinary vanillylmandelic acid	H	Short adrenocorticotropic hormone stimulation test
D	Oral glucose tolerance test with levels of growth hormone	I	Thyroid antibodies
E	Plasma and urine osmolarity	J	Thyroid-stimulating hormone

For each of the following cases, select the single most appropriate endocrinological test. Each option may be used once, more than once or not at all.

4. A 30-year-old man was diagnosed with Cushing's disease.

5. A 32-year-old man was started on olanzapine. After 2 months, he was diagnosed with diabetes mellitus.

6. A 40-year-old woman was diagnosed with a phaeochromocytoma.

7. A 32-year-old man presented with soft-tissue overgrowth, and big jaws, hands and feet.

PSYCHOPHARMACOLOGY: PHARMACODYNAMICS

Theme: Mechanism of side effects of antipsychotics

Options for questions: 8–10

A α_1-adrenergic receptor blockade

B   Asymmetrical σ_1-receptor activation in frontal cortex

C   Decreased density of neuronal nicotinic cholinergic receptors

D   Dopamine D_4-receptor activation in the hippocampus

E   Dopamine receptor super sensitivity

F   High dopamine D_2-receptor occupancy in striatum

G   Low dopamine D_2-receptor occupancy in striatum

For each of the following side effects, select the single most appropriate mechanism. Each option may be used once, more than once or not at all.

8.   Postural hypotension

9.   Parkinsonism

10.   Tardive dyskinesia

PSYCHOPHARMACOLOGY: PHARMACOKINETICS

Theme: Mechanism of action of psychotropic drugs

Options questions: 11–13

A   Amisulpride

B   Aripiprazole

C   Buspirone

D   Chlorpromazine

E   Duloxetine

F   Galantamine

G   Moclobemide

H   Reboxetine

For each of the following mechanisms of action, select the single most appropriate drug. Each option may be used once, more than once or not at all.

11. D_2-Receptor partial agonist

12.   5-Hydroxytryptamine 1A partial agonist

13.   Noradrenaline selective reuptake inhibitor

Theme: Adverse drug reactions of antidepressants

Options for questions: 14–16

A	Citalopram	F	Paroxetine
B	Clomipramine	G	St John's wort
C	Fluroxamine	H	Tranylcypromine
D	Maprotiline	I	Venlafaxine
E	Mirtazapine		

For each of the following descriptions, select the single most appropriate medication. Each option may be used once, more than once or not at all.

14. This drug showed no advantage over selective serotonin reuptake inhibitors (SSRIs) in low doses. It is often used in patients with hypersomnia and atypical presentation of depressive disorder. It has possibly more rapid onset of action than SSRIs, but is poorly tolerated at medium-to-high doses. Withdrawal effects are common.

15. This drug is often used in depressed patients with anxiety and severe sleep disturbance. Sedation may be inversely related to dose prescribed. Its side-effect profile is predominantly histamine 1 (H_1) receptor antagonism.

16. This drug is a potent inhibitor at cytochrome CYP450-2D6 and inhibits its own metabolism. It is well tolerated by patients with panic and mixed anxiety and depressive disorders. Its abrupt withdrawal may cause gastrointestinal disturbance and movement disorders.

Theme: Mechanisms of action of psychotropic drugs

Options for questions: 17–20

A	Agomelatine	F	Milnacipran
B	Atomoxetine	G	Mirtazapine
C	Bupropion	H	Trazodone
D	Buspirone	I	Venlafaxine
E	Duloxetine	J	Ziprasidone

For each of the following mechanisms of action, select the single most appropriate medication that acts via that mechanism. Each option may be used once, more than once or not at all.

17. 5-Hydroxytryptamine 1A (5-HT_{1A}) partial agonist

18. Selective noradrenaline re-uptake inhibitor

19. 5-HT_{2A} antagonist and 5-HT reuptake inhibitor

20. Melatonin receptor agonist

PSYCHOPHARMACOLOGY: ADVERSE REACTIONS

Theme: SSRI-induced side effects

Options for questions: 21–23

A	Stimulation of 5-hydroxytryptamine 2A $(5\text{-}HT_{2A})$ and $5\text{-}HT_{2C}$ in limbic cortex	E	Stimulation of $5\text{-}HT_{2A}$ in mesocortical centres
B	Stimulation of $5\text{-}HT_{2A}$ in basal ganglia	F	Stimulation of $5\text{-}HT_{2A}$ in spinal cord
C	Stimulation of $5\text{-}HT_{2A}$ in brain stem	G	Stimulation of $5\text{-}HT_3$ in basal ganglia
D	Stimulation of $5\text{-}HT_{2A}$ in GI tract	H	Stimulation of $5\text{-}HT_3$ in hypothalamus
		I	Stimulation of $5\text{-}HT_3$ in limbic cortex

For each of the following adverse effects of SSRI drugs, select the single most appropriate explanation of mechanism. Each option may be used once, more than once or not at all.

21. Myoclonus

22. Delayed ejaculation

23. Decreased libido

GENETICS

Theme: Genetic tests and their clinical use

Options for questions: 24–27

A	Chromatin remodelling	G	Quadruple test
B	Guthrie's test	H	Small RNAs
C	Hardy–Weinberg equilibrium		(micro-RNAs, small interfering RNAs)
D	Imprinting genes	I	Southern blotting technique
E	Phenotypic equilibrium	J	Western blotting test
F	Polymerised chain reaction		

For each of the following descriptions, select the single most appropriate genetic test. Each option may be used once, more than once or not at all.

24. Nucleosomes in the DNA have dynamic properties, thus affecting the transcription. It is a form of epigenetic modification of DNA.

25. A screening test to be done in a newborn who later presented with a learning disability, microcephaly, epilepsy, fair hair and skin, eczema, hyperactivity and autistic features.

26. This test has serum inhibin-A assay as its component.

27. This test is associated with cognitive dysfunction.

Theme: Genes involved in schizophrenia

Options for questions: 28–30

A COMT
B DAOA
C DISC1
D DISC2

E PRODH2
F Dysbindin
G Neuregulin

For each of the following chromosome locations, select the single most appropriate gene that is situated at this location. Each option may be used once, more than once or not at all.

28. Chromosome 1q42.1

29. Chromosome 6p22.3

30. Chromosome 8p21-22

Theme: Authors associated with terminology in genetics

Options for questions: 31–34

A DNA
B Gene
C Genetics
D Genome

E Genotype
F Nucleus
G Polygene
H RNA

For each of the following authors, select the terminology/terminologies with which he or she is associated according to further instructions. Each option may be used once, more than once or not at all.

31. GK Mather (select ONE options)

32. Maurice Wilkins (select ONE option)

33. Wilhelm Johannsen (select TWO options)

34. William Bateson (select ONE option)

EPIDEMIOLOGY: SURVEYS ACROSS LIFE SPAN AND MEASURES

Theme: Statistical tests in clinical research

Options for questions: 35–37

A Angoff's method
B Area under the curve
C Bonferroni's method
D Likelihood ratio

E Mann–Whitney U-test
F Receiver operating characteristic curve
G Tchaikovsky's method
H The paired t-test

For each of the following descriptions, select the single most appropriate term that best describes it. Each option may be used once, more than once or not at all.

35. This method is used to identify the best compromise between sensitivity and specificity of a test.

36. This process is used when a number of hypothesis are being evaluated using p values.

37. In this approach, a group of experts are consulted to obtain a raw cut score.

Theme: Sampling methods in clinical research

Options for questions: 38–40

A	Cluster sampling	E	Simple sampling
B	Progressive sampling	F	Snowball sampling
C	Quota sampling	G	Stratified sampling
D	Random sampling	H	Systemic sampling

For each of the following descriptions, select the single most appropriate sampling method. Each option may be used once, more than once or not at all.

38. Every twentieth name on a school admission list

39. To determine rates of depression in white and Asian people

40. To determine rates of schizophrenia in black ethnic and illegal immigrants

ADVANCED PSYCHOLOGICAL PROCESSES AND TREATMENTS

Theme: Normative and non-normative shifts

Options for questions: 41–43

A	Being employed	H	Increasing autonomy and responsibility
B	Bereavement	I	Learning a foreign language
C	Receiving an award in school	J	Menarche
D	Getting a driving licence	K	Parental divorce
E	Growth spurt	L	Physical strength
F	Going on holiday	M	Right to vote acquired
G	Illness	N	Self-harm

For each of the following shifts, according to Kloep and Hendry, select the most appropriate transition/transitions as per further instructions. Each option may be used once, more than once or not at all.

41. Normative society-dependent shift (select TWO options).

42. Normative maturational shift (select THREE options).

43. Non-normative shift (select THREE options).

Theme: Effects of family adversities

Options for questions: 44–46

A Child abuse is more common
B Child has negative peer interactions even before separation
C There is an established causal link to developing a psychotic illness in adulthood
D There is a higher prevalence in children reared by homosexual couples
E School performance is usually unaffected
F Sons are usually compliant to mothers
G The relationship between mother and daughter is affected in mothers who do not remarry
H There are links to adolescent criminal behaviour
I Weight loss is usually the first indicator of adversity

For each of the following family adversities, select the single most appropriate effect associated with it. Each option may be used once, more than once or not at all.

44. Marital conflict

45. Lone parents

46. Childhood physical abuse

Theme: Therapy models in children and adolescents

Options for questions: 47–48

A Art therapy
B Cognitive–behavioural therapy
C Eye-movement desensitisation and reprocessing
D Desensitisation
E Play therapy
F Psychodynamic psychotherapy
G Systemic family therapy

For each of the following cases, select the single most appropriate intervention. Each option may be used once, more than once or not at all.

47. A 12-year-old boy presented with problems in childhood that resulted from inappropriate family structure and organisation.

48. A 14-year-old adolescent girl presented with depression.

Answers: EMIs

1. C Amnesia

Amnesia is defined as memory impairment after a brain injury, neurological illness, or iatrogenic or psychological trauma. Individuals with amnesia may have normal short-term or immediate memory. Lesion in either side of basal forebrain can give rise anterograde, retrograde amnesia and confabulation.

2. A Acquired sociopathy

Individuals with acquired sociopathy can present with memory impairement, lack of concern, disinhibited behaviour and lability of mood. Acquired sociopathy is also known as pseudo-psychopathic disorder. Lesion in either side of the orbital cortex can give rise to acquired sociopathy.

3. F Dysprosody

A lesion in the non-dominant (right-side) areas 44 and 45 can give rise to dysprosody (**Table 6.1**).

Table 6.1 Dysprosody	
Localisation of lesion	**Condition**
Broca's area; dominant side: 44 and 45	Expressive aphasia (motor)
Broca's area; non-dominant side: 44 and 45	Dysprosody
Superior mesial region (either side)	Akinetic mutism
Orbital cortex (either side)	Acquired sociopathy
Basal forebrain (either side)	Anterograde and retrograde amnesia and confabulation
Wernicke's area–superior temporal gyrus–posterior part–area 22 (left)	Receptive aphasia (sensory)
Posterior part of middle, inferior and fourth temporal gyrus and adjoining occipitotemporal junction	Prosopagnosia
Anterior part of middle, inferior and fourth temporal gyrus and temporal pole on the left side	Anomia

4. A Dexamethasone suppression test

Cushing's syndrome is caused by hypercortisolism. In this condition patients may present with comorbid neuropsychiatric symptoms and signs of depression, psychosis, mania and confusion. The dexamethasone suppression test is used to demonstrate the continued production of endogenous cortisol despite the administration of an exogenous steroid.

5. B Fasting plasma glucose

Second-generation antipsychotic medication is associated with metabolic syndrome. It can cause an alteration in blood glucose levels and could be responsible for causing diabetes mellitus. The most useful test to diagnose diabetes mellitus is a fasting plasma glucose test.

6. C 24-hour urinary VMA

Phaeochromocytoma is one of the rare catecholamine-producing tumours. In this condition, the patient presents with episodic hypertension, anxiety and chest tightness. Glycosuria during the attacks is present in about 30% of patients. A 24-hour urine collection for vanillylmandelic acid is the screening test for diagnosis of a phaeochromocytoma. In addition, metanephrines and catecholamines can also be checked in the plasma for diagnosis.

7. D Oral glucose tolerance test with levels of growth hormone

Acromegaly is a rare disease, which is caused by hypersecretion of growth hormone (GH) from a pituitary tumour. It usually presents between ages of 30 and 50 years. It is characterised by excessive soft-tissue growth. Patients may present with the psychological effects of their disease which include mood swings, low self-esteem, body image distortion, social withdrawal and anxiety. The definite test for diagnosis is the oral glucose tolerance test with GH levels.

In case of diabetes insipidus, patient may present with polyuria, polydipsia, and dehydration. Investigations that are useful to diagnose the condition are urea and electrolytes, calcium, plasma and urine osmolality. Plasma osmolality should be high and urine osmolality should be low in order to assist this diagnosis.

8. A α_1-Adrenergic receptor blockade

Postural hypotension is commonly associated with antipsychotic drugs that are antagonist at postsynaptic adrenergic α_1-receptors. Clozapine, chlorpromazine, quetiapine and risperidone are associated with postural hypotension. In addition, some drugs are antagonists at presynaptic α_2-adrenergic receptors, which can lead to increased release of noradrenaline, increased vagal activity and vasoconstriction.

9. F High dopamine D_2-receptor occupancy in striatum

Parkinsonism results from the antagonistic action of antipsychotics at dopamine D_2-receptors in the basal ganglia including the corpus striatum.

10. E Dopamine receptor supersensitivity

Tardive dyskinesia can present with choreiform, athetoid, dystonic, stereotypic or a combination of these movements. High-risk groups who may develop tardive dyskinesia include women, elderly patients, or someone with an underlying brain disease, mood disorder or diabetes mellitus. Its mechanism is considered to be receptor up-regulation, which is described as an increase in the postsynaptic receptors and supersensitivity due to chronic pharmacological antagonism.

11. B Aripiprazole

This is a partial dopamine agonist with high affinity for dopamine D_2- and D_3-receptors. It has affinity for 5-hydroxytryptamine 1A (5-HT_{1A}) receptors as partial agonist but without much affinity for D_1-receptors. It possesses antagonist affinity for 5-HT_{2A}-, 5-HT_6- and 5-HT_7-receptors.

12. C Buspirone

This is a partial serotonin 5-HT_{1A}- receptor agonist, dopamine D_2- and D_3-receptor agonist, D_4-receptor antagonist and partial $α_1$-receptor agonist. It is used in short- and long-term treatment of generalised anxiety disorder.

13. H Reboxetine

This is a selective noradrenaline reuptake inhibitor. Although weight gain and sedation are unusual with reboxetine, side effects such as β insomnia, anxiety, agitation, sexual dysfunction, dry mouth, urinary retention, hypotension and constipation can occur.

14. I Venlafaxine

This has a dual action on serotonin and noradrenaline receptors. At higher doses it acts in dopamine as well. Its pharmacological properties resemble those of clomipramine to some extent. However, unlike clomipramine and other tricyclic antidepressants, it has a negligible affinity for other neuroreceptor sites. Hence, it lacks sedative and anticholinergic effects.

15. E Mirtazapine

This is an analogue of mianserin and has a similar pharmacological property. However, it has weaker affinity for $α_1$-adrenoreceptors. This permits mirtazapine to activate serotonin as well as noradrenaline-neurons. It is known as a noradrenaline and serotonin-specific antidepressant. It has a sedative profile and can be used in depressed patients with sleep disturbance.

16. F Paroxetine

This is absorbed slowly and its peak plasma level is achieved after 4–8 hours. It has a half-life of 20–30 hours. Extrapyramidal side effects such as parkinsonism and akathisia are more common with selective serotonin reuptake inhibitors than tricyclic antidepressants. In particular, paroxetine is associated with acute dystonias in the first few days of treatment.

17. D Buspirone

This is a short acting 5-HT_{1A} partial agonist which is used for anxiety disorders but not as an anxiolytic. It is administered twice or thrice daily. It is also used in combination with selective serotonin reuptake inhibitors (SSRIs) to augment its action. It would act on somatodendritic 5-HT_{1A} autoreceptors to replete serotonin levels and SSRIs can block 5-HT reuptake. It does not cause sexual dysfunction, unlike SSRIs.

18. B Atomoxetine

Reboxetine and atomoxetine are selective noradrenaline reuptake inhibitors. Atomoxetine is primarily used to treat attention deficit hyperactivity disorder. As a result of selective action, they lack the additional undesirable properties of tricyclic antidepressants. However, for the same reason they are not considered as strong or effective as other agents that have multiple actions.

19. H Trazodone

Trazodone and nefazodone are 5 (5-HT$_{2A}$) antagonist and 5-HT reuptake inhibitors (serotonin antagonist/reuptake inhibitor). They block 5-HT$_{2A}$, 5-HT$_{2C}$ and serotonin transporters. All three mechanisms are responsible for the antidepressant action. They also block α_1-receptors leading to undesirable effects.

20. A Agomelatine

This is a melatonin receptor agonist. It is the first antidepressant that acts on melatonergic receptors. It is a 5-HT$_{2C}$ and 5-HT$_{2B}$ antagonist.

21. C Stimulation of 5-HT$_{2A}$ in the brain stem

SSRIs stimulate 5-HT$_{2A}$ receptors in the brain stem resulting in myoclonus and slow-wave sleep disturbance.

22. F Stimulation of 5-HT$_{2A}$ in the spinal cord

SSRIs are known to cause sexual side effects such as decreased libido, anorgasmia and erectile dysfunction. Stimulation of serotonin and its release in the brain and spinal cord leads to a decrease in noradrenaline and dopamine. This results in sexual side effects including delayed ejaculation.

23. E Stimulation of 5-HT$_{2A}$ in mesocortical centres

The undesirable side effects of SSRIs seem to involve not only specific 5-HT-receptor subtypes but also the action of serotonin at the receptors in specific areas of the body, including the brain, spinal cord and gut. Different side effects and their causation, depending on the receptor subtype and site of action, are mentioned in **Table 6.2**. In a patient treated with SSRIs, who experienced agitation, anxiety, apathy and sexual dysfunction, it could be really difficult to know whether this represents incomplete recovery from depression or the side effects of SSRIs. In this case, adding or switching to a different class of drugs that acts on dopamine, noradrenaline or GABA may be required. Many other antidepressants that act through a separate mechanism have different side-effect profiles. For example, mirtazapine blocks 5-HT$_{2A}$, 5-HT$_{2C}$ and 5-HT$_3$-receptors, and therefore lacks many of the side effects caused by SSRIs. The same applies to nefazodone which blocks 5-HT$_{2A}$.

24. A Chromatin remodelling

DNA is packed in chromatin in a repeat of histone DNA complexes, which are called nucleosomes. DNA has to get rid of the nucleosomes so that it is available for the transcription factors and RNA polymerase for transcription. Nucleosomes have dynamic properties that ultimately affect the transcription and, as with DNA methylation, are heritable and in fact another form of epigenetic modification of DNA. Histones are proteins and present in nucleosomes cores. Chromatin remodelling involves either the movement of the nucleosome along the length of the DNA molecule, a process known as 'nucleosome sliding', or by chromatin remodellers, which cause disruption and reorganisation of the nucleosome core, making the DNA available for transcription.

25. B Guthrie's test

Phenylketonuria is the third most common cause of learning disability after Down's syndrome and fragile X syndrome. It is an autosomal recessive condition and occurs in 1:14,000 live births. There is absence of an enzyme called phenylalanine hydroxylase, which is responsible for the conversion of phenylalanine to tyrosine. Guthrie's test detects β-subtilis, the multiplication of which depends on phenylalanine. It is carried out 6–14 days after birth. The deficiency of phenylalanine hydroxylase can lead to severe learning disabilities and this can be avoided if phenylalanine is excluded from the diet. Sufferers may present with autistic behaviour, cerebral palsy, a characteristic mousy odour, fits, eczema, fair hair, blue eyes, etc.

26. G Quadruple test

This is a screening blood test for Down's syndrome and spina bifida. It can detect women who are at higher risk of their baby having either of these conditions. It cannot tell whether the fetus has or doesn't have Down's syndrome or spina bifida. The test measures four hormones in the blood: α-fetoprotein, β-human chorionic gonadotrophin, inhibin-A and oestriol.

27. D Imprinting genes

Intellectual disabilities that are present in 'imprinting' disorders such as Prader–Willi syndrome, Angelman's syndrome, Rett's and Turner's syndromes are due to imprinting genes.

Hardy–Weinberg equilibrium states that the allele (say if the alleles are either C or T) and genotype (genotypes will be CC, CT, TT) frequencies in a large population remain constant, i.e. in equilibrium in any population over generations in the absence of migration, mutation, assortative mating (or random mating), and natural selection. It is almost impossible that the Hardy–Weinberg equilibrium exists in nature (i.e. not evolving). The importance of the Hardy–Weinberg model is that it enables scientists to compare a change in a population's genetic structure over a period of time. If a population's genetic structure stays in Hardy–Weinberg equilibrium it will indicate a state of 'no evolution'.

28. C DISC 1

This gene is located in chromosome 1q42.1. It encodes for a protein called disrupted in schizophrenia 1. It is implicated in disorders such as schizophrenia, depression and bipolar disorder.

29. F Dysbindin

Dystrobrevin-binding protein-1, also known as dysbindin, is located on chromosome 6p22.3. A strong association has been noticed between dysbindin expression and schizophrenia. Hermansky–Pudlak syndrome type 7 is an autosomal recessive condition that is caused by mutation in the dysbindin gene.

30. G Neuregulin

This is situated on chromosome 8p21-22.

COMT gene is located in chromosome 22q11. DAOA, known as D-amino acid oxidase activator, or G72 is located in 1224.11.

31. G Polygene

GK Mather coined the term 'polygene'. When a certain phenotypic trait is influenced by two or more non-allelic genes, it can lead to polygenic inheritance. Eye colour is determined by two or more genes and hence is polygenic in nature.

32. A DNA

Watson, Crick and Wilkins received the noble prize in physiology or medicine in 1953 for determination of the structure of DNA.

33. B, E Gene. Genotype

Wilhelm Johannsen coined the term 'gene'. He has also coined the terms 'genotype' and phenotype'.

34. C Genetics

William Bateson coined the term 'genetics'.

35. F Receiver operating characteristic curve (ROC)

Theoretically, the most desirable balance between the values of sensitivity and specificity to be possessed by a test can be determined by a lengthy procedure involving measurement of the sensitivity and specificity values at different cut-off points, using a gold standard as reference. The sensitivity and specificity value obtained for cut-off points can also be presented graphically on an ROC. The closest point on the ROC to the ideal state represents the best sensitivity and specificity compromise, and the total area under the curve (AUC) of a test represents the probability of that test correctly identifying true positives and true negatives, i.e. test accuracy.

36. C Bonferroni's method

This method is an example of a closed test procedure. It controls the family-wise error rate for all the K hypotheses. Suppose that there are K new hypotheses each with a p value to be tested and the overall type 1 error rate is α, then all the p values $< \alpha / K$ are rejected.

37. A Angoff's method

In this approach, a group of experts is used to obtain a raw cut score. In this approach, a group of experts are used to obtain a raw cut score. It is a study that is used by examination or test setters to determine a cut-off for pass and fail results. The Royal College of Psychiatrists uses Angoff's method to set a standard for pass marks for theory papers 1, 2 and 3.

By combining the sensitivity and specificity values of a test, a more versatile and readily applicable measure of test validity may be derived. This measure is called a likelihood ratio and can be calculated for every possible result category of a test. It is a measure of the probability of a test result being seen in an individual with a disorder relative to it being seen in an unaffected individual.

38. H Systematic sampling

A random sample of the whole population should represent the whole population. The systematic sample involves arranging the target population according to some ordering scheme and then selecting elements at regular intervals through that ordered list.

39. G Stratified sampling

This is the process of dividing members of the population into homogeneous subgroups before sampling and, for example, it is used for culture and racial studies.

40. F Snowballing sampling

This method recruits future participants from among their acquaintances. In other words, the sample group appears to grow like a rolling snowball. Cluster sampling is used when natural groupings are evident in a studied population.

41. D, M Getting a driving licence. Right to vote acquired

The shifts involved in a transition can be captured as 'normative' and 'non-normative' shifts. These were described by Hendry and Kloep in 1999.

42. E, H, J Growth spurt. Increasing autonomy and responsibility. Menarche

The normative maturational shift includes physical and cognitive changes that occur during adolescence in the individual, e.g. menarche, growth spurt, voice breaking and becoming more independent. The normative society-dependent shift includes transitions that occur in the environment around the individual, e.g. acquiring the right to vote and moving from primary to high school, starting an occupation (not merely being employed) and getting a licence to drive.

43. B, G, K Bereavement. Illness. Parental divorce

The non-normative shifts include changes to which the individual is subjected to as a result of adversity and self or the environment, e.g. parental divorce, illness, physical/learning disability or bereavement.

44. B Child has negative peer interactions even before separation

The effects of marital conflict are seen on children even before divorce or separation. The children are likely to have more stress and negative peer interactions. The effects on the child vary depending on the age of the child at the time of divorce or separation. The relationship between the mother and son is affected in mothers who do not remarry. There are no similar findings between the mother–daughter relationships. Sons are usually non-compliant to mother's control.

45. A Child abuse is more common

Child abuse occurs more commonly with lone parents. The effects of childhood physical abuse include adolescent criminal behaviour and violence as an adult (familial and non-familial). Childhood sexual abuse can have long-term effects on mental health.

46. H There are links to adolescent criminal behaviour

Evidence suggests clear links to criminal behaviour in this situation. Research to date on children reared by homosexual couples does not show that the children develop significantly differently in any way.

47. G Systemic family therapy

Salvador Minuchin developed systemic family therapy, in the 1960s. It looks at structure and subsystems within the family. Therapy focuses on action more than insight and is based on normative family models with clear boundaries and hierarchies. The therapy views the presentation of the problems of the child as a result of dysfunction within the family system.

48. B Cognitive–behavioural therapy

In depression, cognitive approaches in children and adolescents are useful to restructure cognitions, improve social skills and improve self-control skills. There is evidence from randomised controlled studies to support the use of this counselling or no treatment.

Chapter 7

Test questions: 2

Questions: EMIs

NEUROSCIENCES: NEUROANATOMY

Theme: Blood supply of brain

Options for questions: 1–4

A   Anterior cerebral artery
B   Anterior choroidal artery
C   Anterior inferior cerebellar artery
D   Basilar artery
E   Middle cerebral artery

F   Posterior cerebral artery
G   Recurrent artery of Heubner
H   Superior cerebellar artery
I   Vertebral artery

For each of the following areas of brain, select the most appropriate artery/arteries that supply them according to further instructions. Each option may be used once, more than once or not at all.

1. Anterior limb of internal capsule (select TWO options)

2. Posterior limb of internal capsule (select TWO options)

3. Basal ganglia (select THREE options)

4. Head of caudate nucleus (select ONE option)

NEUROSCIENCES: NEUROPATHOLOGY

Theme: Dementia and gene/chromosome

Options for questions: 5–8

A   Dementia of Lewy bodies
B   Down's syndrome dementia
C   Huntington's disease
D   Familial Alzheimer's dementia

E   Progressive supranuclear palsy
F   Sporadic Alzheimer's dementia
G   Sporadic Creutzfeldt-Jakob disease
H   Variant Creutzfeldt-Jakob disease

For each of the following genes/chromosomes, select the single most appropriate diagnosis that is associated with it. Each option may be used once, more than once or not at all.

5. APP and $ApoeE_4$.

6. Mutation in chromosome 14 and chromosome 1

7. Mutation in tau modulating genes

8. Mutation in chromosome 4

PSYCHOPHARMACOLOGY: PHARMACODYNAMICS

Theme: Termination of action of neurotransmitters

Options for questions: 9–13

A Breakdown by catechol-O-methyltransferase (COMT) and decarboxylase
B Breakdown by COMT and monoamine oxidase A (MAO-A)
C Breakdown by COMT and MAO-B
D Breakdown by hydroxylase and decarboxylase
E Breakdown by MAO-A and decarboxylase
F Breakdown by MAO-A and MAO-B
G Breakdown by MAO-A, MAO-B and COMT
H Breakdown by MAO-B and hydroxylase
I Breakdown by transaminase
J No enzymatic breakdown responsible for terminating the action

For each of the following neurotransmitters, select the single most appropriate mechanism responsible for termination of their action. Each option may be used once, more than once or not at all.

9. Dopamine

10. Hydroxytryptamine

11. Noradrenaline

12. Aminobutyric acid (GABA)

13. Glutamate

PSYCHOPHARMACOLOGY: ADVERSE REACTIONS

Theme: Pharmacology of adverse effects of drugs

Options for questions: 14–17

A Anti-adrenergic activity
B Antihistaminergic activity
C Antimuscarinic activity
D Cholinergic activity
E Decreased serotoninergic activity
F Increased dopaminergic activity
G Increased adrenergic activity
H Increased serotoninergic activity

For each of the following adverse effects, select the single most appropriate mechanism. Each option may be used once, more than once or not at all.

14. Akathisia

15. Weight gain

16. Prolonged erection

17. Hyperthermia

PSYCHOPHARMACOLOGY: PHARMACODYNAMICS

Theme: Chemical classification of antipsychotics

Options for questions: 18–21

A Aripiprazole	F Pimozide
B Chlorpromazine	G Quetiapine
C Clozapine	H Risperidone
D Haloperidol	I Sulpiride
E Olanzapine	J Zuclopenthixol

For each of the following chemical class, select the single most appropriate antipsychotic drug that is classified under that class. Each option may be used once, more than once or not at all.

18. Benzisoxazole

19. Dibenzithiezepine

20. Quinolinone

21. Thienobenzodiazepine

PSYCHOPHARMACOLOGY: PHARMACODYNAMICS

Theme: Interaction of sodium valproate with other drugs

Options for questions: 22–25

A Amitriptyline	F Lamotrigine
B Carbamazepine	G Oral contraceptives
C Diazepam	H Phenobarbital
D Fluoxetine	I Phenytoin
E Folic acid	

For each of the following drug interactions, select the most appropriate drug/drugs involved according to further instructions. Each option may be used once, more than once or not at all.

22. Serum concentration of this drug is decreased by valproate (select ONE option).

23. Serum concentration of these drugs is increased by valproate (select THREE options).

24. Serum concentration of valproate is decreased by this drug (select ONE option).

25. Serum concentration of valproate is increased by these drugs (select TWO options).

Theme: Half-life of psychotropic drugs in hours

Options for questions: 26–29

A	1 hour	E	5–15 hours	
B	2 hours	F	10 hours	
C	3 hours	G	20–100 hours	
D	4 hours	H	24 hours	

For each of the following drugs, select the single most appropriate half-life. Each option may be used once, more than once or not at all.

26. Alprazolam

27. Flurazepam

28. Diazepam

29. Zaleplon

GENETICS

Theme: Genetic tests and their associations

Options for questions: 30–33

A	Chromatin remodelling	G	Quadruple test	
B	Guthrie test	H	Small RNAs (micro-RNAs, small interfering RNAs)	
C	Hardy–Weinberg equilibrium			
D	Imprinting genes	I	Southern blotting technique	
E	Northern blotting technique	J	Western blot test	
F	Polymerised chain reaction			

For each of the following descriptions, select the single most appropriate genetic test. Each option may be used once, more than once or not at all.

30. A technique used for detection of mRNA

31. A technique wherein a genomic DNA is cut down into fragments by a restriction enzyme and is then separated into DNA fragments of different sizes by gel and electrophoresis

32. A technique implicated in post-transcriptional gene repression

33. A technique that allows us to amplify a single or a few copies of a piece of DNA against a background of a large excess of irrelevant DNA

Theme: Genetical disorders

Options for questions: 34–37

A   Chromosome 11
B   Hurler's syndrome
C   Klinefelter's syndrome
D   Myotonic dystrophy
E   Phenylketonuria

F   Rett's syndrome
G   Sturge–Weber syndrome
H   Tay–Sachs disease
I   Velocardiofacial syndrome
J   Xq27

For each of the following signs or symptoms, select the single most appropriate diagnosis. Each option may be used once, more than once or not at all.

34. Attention deficit hyperactivity disorder

35. Angiomas

36. Aniridia

37. Cleft palate

Theme: Genes and psychiatric conditions

Options for questions: 38–40

A   *5-HTTLPR* gene
B   *BDNF* gene
C   COMT gene
D   *CREB* gene

E   Dopamine transporter gene
F   *SLITRK-1* gene
G   Tryptophan hydroxylase 1 gene

For each of the following psychiatric conditions, select the single most appropriate gene associated with it. Each option may be used once, more than once or not at all.

38. Quantitative risk factor for suicidal behaviour

39. Impulsive and aggressive personality traits

40. Gilles de la Tourette's syndrome in white population

Theme: Genetic processes

Options for questions: 41–44

A   Crossing over
B   Dislocation
C   Modification
D   Mutations

E   Transcription
F   Transformation
G   Translation
H   Translocation

For each of the following descriptions, select the single most appropriate genetic process that describes it best. Each option may be used once, more than once or not at all.

41. The process by which genetic material between homologous chromosomes gets exchanged

42. The process by which genetic material between non-homologous chromosomes gets exchanged

43. The process by which genetic material within a chromosome changes

44. The process by which the information from DNA is converted to mRNA

ADVANCED PSYCHOLOGICAL PROCESSES AND TREATMENTS: PERSONALITY DISORDERS

Theme: Diagnosis of the ICD-10 personality disorders

Options for questions: 45–47

A   Anankastic personality disorder
B   Anxious–avoidant personality disorder
C   Dependent personality disorder
D   Dissocial personality disorder

E   Emotionally unstable personality disorder
F   Histrionic personality disorder
G   Paranoid personality disorder
H   Schizoid personality disorder

For each of the following cases, select the single most appropriate diagnosis. Each option may be used once, more than once or not at all.

45. A 34-year-old woman complained of feeling uneasy almost every day. She went out only with her older sister, whom she thought was better liked by everyone. She preferred her sister to be with her because she believed that she was likely to be criticised by others for frivolous things and will need her sister to speak up for her.

46. A 28-year-old woman had been estranged from her family due to being unpredictable and always getting into trouble throughout her life. Her mother had a history of being abused by her various partners, and she had never known her father. She had on occasions presented to the mental health services for hearing voices and feeling suspicious of other people. She had received treatment for depression and had on occasion needed admission to the acute assessment unit for attempts at self-harm, usually precipitated by personal crises.

47. A 41-year-old man had always been a loner. He appeared not to be bothered by criticism from his colleagues, who felt that, despite several attempts, 'he just did not fit in'. He was quite introspective, and was exceptionally good at his job and dealing with numbers.

Theme: Prevalence of personality disorders

Options for questions: 48–50

A   As high as 15% in inpatient settings
B   As high as 20% in inpatient settings
C   As high as 30% in inpatient settings
D   Equality in males and females
E   Less frequent in inpatient settings

F   More common in females than males
G   Most common in the general population
H   More frequent in inpatient settings than the community
I   More common in males

For each of the following personality disorders, select two most appropriate options. Each option may be used once, more than once or not at all.

48. Paranoid personality disorder

49. Dependent personality disorder

50. Anxious–avoidant personality disorder

EPIDEMIOLOGY

Theme: Practical application of descriptive statistics

Options for questions: 51–54

A	Cumulative incidence	E	Lifetime prevalence
B	Incidence	F	Period prevalence
C	Isolated incidence	G	Point prevalence
D	Lateral prevalence	H	Proportional morbidity

For each of the following definitions, select the single most appropriate terminology that best describes it. Each option may be used once, more than once or not at all.

51. This measure is defined as the frequency of a disease during a period of time in all the individuals in the population at risk.

52. This is a measure of the total number of cases in the population, divided by the number of individuals in the population on a given day.

53. This is a measure of the total number of individuals with a disease over a 1-year period in a circumscribed population.

54. This is the number of individuals in a statistical population who at some point in their life had experienced an illness, compared with the total number of individuals.

Theme: Psychotherapy techniques

Options for questions: 55–58

A	Cognitive restructuring	F	Holding
B	Competing interests and habit reversal	G	Mindfulness
C	Dream interpretation	H	Parapraxis
D	Exposure and response prevention	I	Positive reinforcement
E	Extinction	J	Relabelling

For each of the following cases, select the single most appropriate therapy. Each option may be used once, more than once or not at all.

55. Parents of a 10-year-old boy reported that they were unable to manage his aggressive behaviour. They were separated and were going through a difficult divorce. The parents did not communicate with each other except when they discussed his behaviour.

56. A 13-year-old girl had a fear of germs. She was observed to be washing her hands several times a day and this had impaired her daily functioning. She had developed dermatitis from repeatedly washing her hands.

57. A 14-year-old boy suffered with low mood and believed that he was a failure at school because he did badly on a test. He also felt that the other children did not like him because they did not call him out to play every weekend. He no longer enjoyed activities that he had previously enjoyed. His development until 3 months ago was unremarkable.

58. A 7-year-old boy had vocal and motor tics that had been present for 18 months. They wax and wane and disturb his home and school life.

Answers: EMIs

1. C, E Anterior inferior cerebellar artery. Middle cerebral artery

The internal capsule is divided into three parts: anterior, genu and posterior internal.

The superior half of the anterior capsule, genu and superior half of the posterior capsule are supplied by the lenticular branch of the middle cerebral artery. The inferior half of the anterior internal capsule is supplied by the recurrent artery of Huebner, a branch of the anterior cerebral artery.

2. C, B Anterior inferior cerebellar artery. Anterior choroidal artery

The superior half of the posterior capsule is supplied by the lenticular branch of the middle cerebral artery. The inferior half of the posterior internal capsule is supplied by the anterior choroidal artery, a branch of the internal carotid artery.

3. A, B, C Anterior cerebral artery. Anterior choroidal artery. Anterior inferior cerebellar artery

The blood supply of basal ganglia is largely derived from the lenticulostriate branch of the middle cerebral artery, anterior choroidal artery and anterior cerebral artery.

4. G Recurrent artery of Huebner

The caudate nucleus is divided into three parts: the head, body and tail. The recurrent artery of Huebner, a branch of the anterior cerebral artery, serves the head of caudate. The tail is served by the anterior choroidal artery.

The corpus callosum receives its blood supply from the pericallosal artery (also called arteria pericallosa) which is a branch of the anterior cerebral artery.

5. F Sporadic Alzheimer's dementia

In addition, it also has tau.

6. D Familial Alzheimer's dementia

Mutations are seen in amyloid precursor protein (APP, chromosome 21), presenilin 1 (chromosome 14) and presenilin 2 (chromosome 1)

7. E Progressive supranuclear palsy

Progressive supranuclear palsy has tau polymorphism (chromosome 17) and mutation in tau-modulating gene.

8. C Huntington's disease

This shows mutation in the huntington gene (chromosome 4).

Dementia of Lewy bodies: α-synuclein (chromosome 4)

Down syndrome dementia: Triple gene APP (chromosome 21)

Sporadic Creutzfeldt–Jakob disease: prion gene (PRNP, chromosome 20), codon 129 methionine or valine homozygous)

Variant Creutzfeldt–Jakob disease: prion gene (PRNP, chromosome 20), codon 129 methionine homozygous).

9. G Breakdown by MAO-A, MAO-B and COMT

Dopamine is broken by COMT (extracellular) and MAO-A and MAO-B, which are present in mitochondria.

10. F Breakdown by MAO-A and MAO-B

5-HT, also known as serotonin, is metabolised by MAO into an inactive metabolite. Serotoninergic neurons themselves contain MAO-B, which has low affinity for 5-HT; therefore much of the 5-HT is thought to be degraded by MAO-A outside the neuron once it has been released.

11. G Breakdown by MAO-A, MAO-B and COMT

Noradrenaline is broken down by COMT (extracellular) and MAO-A and MAO-B, which are present in mitochondria.

12. I Breakdown by transaminase

GABA's action is terminated by GABA transaminase (GABA-T), which converts GABA into an inactive substance.

13. J No enzymatic breakdown is responsible for terminating the action

Glutamate is a major excitatory neurotransmitter that is synthesised from glutamine in glial cells. After its release into synapses, it is taken up by neighbouring glial cells by an excitatory amino acid transporter (EAAT). Inside these glial cells, glutamate is converted into glutamine by glutamine synthetase; however, this glutamine is again converted into glutamate by glutaminase. Therefore, once released, glutamate's actions are stopped not by enzymatic breakdown as other neurotransmitters, but by removal by EAATs on neurons or glia and the whole cycle is restarted again.

Hydroxylase converts tryptophan into 5-hydroxytryptophan and then decarboxylase coverts it into serotonin. Another hydroxylase converts tyrosine into dopa, which is converted by decarboxylase into dopamine. In noradrenergic neurons, dopamine is converted into noradrenaline by β-hydroxylase. Another decarboxylase (glutamic acid decarboxylase) synthesises γ-aminobutyric acid from glutamate. Therefore hydroxylase and decarboxylase are used for synthesis of these neurotransmitters, not their termination.

14. H Increased serotoninergic activity

Akathisia is a side effect of the selective serotonin reuptake inhibitors due to excessive serotoninergic activity. Acute stimulation of 5-HT_{2A} receptors in serotoninergic projections of the basal ganglia can lead to inhibition of dopamine transmission which in turn may lead to akathisia and other mild parkinsonian symptoms and agitation. Antipsychotics can also cause akathisia but by directly blocking dopamine receptors.

15. B Antihistaminergic activity

H_1-receptor blockade is mainly responsible for weight gain. It also causes sedation. 5-HT_{2C}-receptor blockade also contributes to weight gain but less than H_1-receptor blockade. Therefore those psychotropics that block H_1-receptors have weight gain as their major side effect, e.g. clozapine, olanzapine, mirtazapine. These drugs have sedative properties for the same reason. It also explains the strong sedating properties of trazodone.

16. A Anti-adrenergic activity

Prolonged erection, also known as priapism, is a prolonged painful erection of the penis not related to any sexual activity or arousal. It can be due to anti-adrenergic activity of α-blocker medications such as prazosin, trazodone. One of the treatments of priapism is injecting α agonists into the penis so as to prevent vascular damage that may lead to penile necrosis.

17. C Antimuscarinic activity

Anticholinergic (or antimuscarinic) activity is responsible for decreased sweating, which in turn may cause hyperthermia. Therefore, overdose (or poisoning) of anticholinergic drugs can present as hyperthermia. Tricyclics have strong anticholinergic properties. Other common side effects of this property are a dry mouth, constipation, blurred vision, narrow angle glaucoma, delirium, etc.

18. H Risperidone

This is a second-generation antipsychotic drug and is a D_2-, 5-HT_{2A}-, α_1-adrenoreceptor and H_1-receptor antagonist agent.

19. G Quetiapine

This is a second-generation antipsychotic drug and is a D_1-, D_2-, 5-HT_{2A}-, α_1-adrenoreceptor and H_1-receptor antagonist agent.

20. A Aripiprazole

This is an interesting compound and it is a D_2-receptor partial agonist with weak 5-HT_{1A}-receptor partial agonism and 5-HT_{2A}-receptor antagonism. It causes nausea and unlike most other antipsychotic agents reduces prolactin levels.

21. E Olanzapine

This is a second-generation antipsychotic drug with D_1-, D_2-, D_4-, 5-HT-, H1- and muscarinic receptor antagonism.

Chlorpromazine is a phenothiazine with an aliphatic side chain.

Haloperidol is a butyrophenone.

Clozapine is a dibenzodiazepine; pimozide belongs to the class called diphenyl butylpiperidine and sulpiride is a substituted benzamide.

Zuclopenthixol is a thioxanthine.

22. I Phenytoin

Valproate decreases the serum concentration of phenytoin due to competition for protein-binding sites. It increases the serum concentration of lamotrigine by decreasing the metabolism (glucuronidation).

23. C, E, H Diazepam. Folic acid. Phenobarbital

This increases the concentration of diazepam by competing for the protein-binding sites. It reduces non-renal clearance of phenobarbital and hence increases the levels.

24. B Carbamazepine

This induces enzymes and hence decreases the levels of sodium valproate.

25. A, D Amitriptyline. Fluoxetine

Amitriptyline and fluoxetine increase the levels of sodium valproate.

26. E 5–15 hours

27. B 2 hours

28. G 20–100 hours

29. A 1 hour

Many benzodiazepines undergo first-pass metabolism and have active metabolites that generally have a much longer elimination half-life than the parent drug. It leads to a prolonged effect and these drugs are generally responsible for a hangover effect or confusion in older age. Benzodiazepines reduce the REM sleep from 10% to 25% of total sleep time. On developing tolerance, REM is normalised (**Table 7.1**).

Table 7.1 Half-lives of benzodiazepines

	Half-life (hours)	Active metabolite half-life (hours)
Alprazolam	5–15	
Diazepam	20–100	30–90
Flurazepam	2	30–100
Lorazepam	10–20	
Nitrazepam	24	30–90
Temazepam	10	
Zaleplon	1	
Zolpidem	2	
Zopiclone	4	3–6

30. E Northern blotting technique

This is used in molecular biology research to study gene expression by detection of RNA (or isolated mRNA) in a sample.

31. I Southern blotting technique

This is used for detection of a specific DNA sequence in DNA samples. DNA fragments are separated by electrophoresis and then transferred to a filter membrane by a blotting procedure, and subsequent fragment detection by a radioactively labelled DNA probe (probe hybridisation). The inventor of this method was a British biologist, Edwin Southern.

32. H Small mRNAs (micro-RNAs, small interfering RNAs)

Small RNAs include micro-RNAs (miRNAs) and small interfering RNAs (siRNAs) alter gene transcription. Th siRNAs can lead to transcriptional silencing. The miRNAs are responsible for post-transcriptional gene repression by base pairing to the message of protein-coding genes.

33. F Polymerase chain reaction

Polymerase chain reaction (PCR) is a technique that enables scientists to amplify a single or a few copies of a piece of DNA of interest against a background of a large excess of irrelevant DNA. It uses oligonucleotide primers which are used to prime DNA synthesis using a heat-stable DNA polymerase.

34. J Xq27

X-linked recessive, fragile X syndrome, also called Martin–Bell syndrome, occurs in 1:1000 of the male population. The fragile site is Xq27 and there is a high possibility of attention deficit disorder and autistic disorder, a variable degree of learning disability, flexible joints, and large ears, chin and testicles. Females are usually carriers but they can also present with features and have learning disability.

35. G Sturge–Weber syndrome

Sturge–Weber syndrome (autosomal dominant) is encephalofacial angiomatosis and around 50% of people with this syndrome have learning disability and epilepsy is common. There are also parieto-occipital intracranial angiomas which can become calcified the and cutaneous naevus distribution on the site of the trigeminal nerve ipsilateral to the angioma.

36. C Klinefelter's syndrome

In Wilms' tumour there is a deletion of chromosome 11 and it presents with aniridia, reduced IQ and ambiguous genitalia.

37. I Velocardiofacial syndrome

This is inherited as autosomal dominant. Approximately a quarter of patients with velocardiofacial syndrome (VCFS) develop psychotic symptoms. This syndrome is denoted as a 22q11.2 deletion syndrome and includes VCFS and DiGeorge's syndrome. Offspring of an individual with 22q11.2 deletion syndrome have a 50% chance of inheriting the 22q11.2 deletion. Psychotic and affective symptoms sometimes do emerge in adolescence or early adulthood. Overall, the prevalence of schizophrenia in VCFS is 25 times more than in the general population. The psychosis associated with VCFS usually runs a chronic course and exhibits a poor response to antipsychotic treatment. VCFS is typically characterised by cleft palate (commonest syndrome associated with cleft palate), cardiac abnormalities and mild learning disabilities.

38. G Tryptophan hydroxylase 1 gene

Two genes have emerged as being involved in vulnerability to suicidality. Tryptophan hydroxylase 1 gene is a quantitative risk factor for suicidal behaviour.

39. A 5-HTTLPR

Serotonin transporter gene (5-HTTLPR) is consistently associated with impulsive, aggressive personality traits.

40. F, G SLITRK-1 gene. Tryptophan hydroxylase 1 gene

Gilles de la Tourette's syndrome shows genetic heterogeneity. However, on rare occasions mutation in the SLITRK-1 gene is associated with Gilles de la Tourette's syndrome in white populations. The SLITRK-1 gene is located on chromosome 13 and is associated with making of SLITRK-1 protein which has a role in nerve cell transmission by influencing growth of specific axons and dendrites.

41. A Crossing over

The process by which the genetic recombination takes place during meiosis is called crossing over. This occurs between homologous chromosomes.

42. G Translation

Sometimes the exchange of genetic material can occur between non-homologous chromosomes. This is called translocation. Translocation can be balanced or non-balanced. It is also called robertsonian or non-robertsonian translocation.

43. D Mutations

This is processes by which changes in genes take place.

44. E Transcription

The process by which information from DNA is converted to mRNA is called transcription.

45. B Anxious–avoidant personality disorder

The case scenario is consistent with a diagnosis of an anxious–avoidant personality disorder. In this disorder, patients consistently feel that they are being criticised by others and feel rejected in social situations. As a result, they avoid situations and relationships that may result in such feelings. They have continuous feeling of tension and anxiety and believe that they are socially inadequate.

46. E Emotionally unstable personality disorder

This case scenario is consistent with the diagnosis of an emotionally unstable personality disorder. In this disorder, the patient can act impulsively without thinking about the consequences. The patient may have mood fluctuation and be unable to carry out any action that may not produce any immediate rewards.

47. H Schizoid personality disorder

The ICD-10 criteria for anxious–avoidant personality disorder include: persistent and pervasive feelings of tension and apprehension, belief that one is socially inept, preoccupation with being criticised and rejected in social situations, and avoidance of activities that involve interpersonal relationships.

Diagnostic features on emotionally unstable personality disorder include: tendency to act unexpectedly and without consideration of the consequences, unstable and capricious mood, difficulty in maintaining any course of action that offers no immediate reward, and a tendency to quarrelsome behaviour.

Diagnostic features of schizoid personality disorder include: few activities provide pleasure, emotional coldness, limited capacity to express warm feelings and choice of solitary activities.

48. C, I As high as 30% in inpatient settings. More common in males

The prevalence of paranoid personality disorder in an inpatient setting is as high as 30%, with it occurring more frequently in males.

49. D, G Equality in males and females. Most common in the general population

Dependent personality disorders occur just as commonly in males and females with an increased occurrence in the general population compared with inpatient settings.

50. D, G Equality in males and females. Most common in the general population

Anxious–avoidant personality disorders such as dependent personality disorder occur just as commonly in both males and females, with an increased occurrence in the general population compared with inpatient settings.

51. A Cumulative incidence

Cumulative incidence is defined as frequency of a disease during a period of time in all the individuals in the population at risk.

52. G Point prevalence

Point prevalence is a measure of the total number of cases in the population, divided by the number of individuals in the population on a given day.

53. F Period prevalence

Period prevalence is a measure of the total number of individuals with a disease over a 1-year period in a circumscribed population.

54. E Lifetime prevalence

Lifetime prevalence is a number of individuals in a statistical population who at some point in their life have experienced an illness, compared with the total number of individuals. Proportional morbidity is the proportion of all individuals with an illness compared with all ill people.

55. J Relabeling

In this case, presentation is related to family dysfunction and managed with systemic family therapy (see **Table 7.2**).

56. D Exposure and response prevention

In this case, a 13-year-old girl has obsessive–compulsive disorder and the psychological intervention involves using exposure and response prevention. Here the fear is confronted while preventing escape behaviours with relaxation training.

57. A Cognitive restructuring

A 14-year-old boy is depressed with cognitive distortions and negative automatic thoughts that are managed by CBT which involves cognitive restructuring along with behavioural interventions and tasks.

58. B Competing interests and habit reversal

A 7-year-old boy has Gilles de la Tourette's syndrome. The psychological intervention employs the technique of competing interest and habit reversal. Usually psychoeducation is the first line of management, as most patients will improve during adolescence.

Dream interpretation, holding and parapraxis are used in psychodynamic therapies.

Extinction and positive reinforcement are behavioural interventions employed in parenting interventions.

Mindfulness is developed in DBT.

Chapter 8

Test questions: 3

Questions: EMIs

NEUROSCIENCES: NEUROENDOCRINOLOGY

Theme: Endocrine tests

Options for questions: 1–5

A   Dexamethasone suppression test
B   Fasting plasma glucose
C   24-hour urinary vanillylmandelic acid
D   Oral glucose tolerance test with levels of growth hormone
E   Plasma and urine osmolarity

F   Plasma aldosterone and renin measurement
G   Parathyroid hormone
H   Short adrenocorticotrophic hormone stimulation test
I   Thyroid antibodies
J   Thyroid-stimulating hormone

For each of the following cases, select the single most appropriate test. Each option may be used once, more than once or not at all.

1.   A 42-year-old man presented with Conn's syndrome.

2.   A 34-year-old woman presented with features of hypocalcaemia.

3.   A 40-year-old man was diagnosed with Addison's disease.

4.   A 45-year-old woman was diagnosed with Graves' disease.

5.   A 30-year-old woman was diagnosed with depression secondary to hypothyroidism.

Theme: Ocular palsies

Options for questions: 6–8

A   Internuclear ophthalmoplegia
B   Lateral gaze palsy
C   Single cranial nerve palsy (III, IV or VI)

D   Skew deviation
E   Supranuclear palsy
F   Vertical gaze palsy

For each of the following lesions, select the single most appropriate palsy. Each option may be used once, more than once or not at all.

6.   A 50-year-old man was diagnosed with a brain-stem lesion.

7.   A 67-year-old woman was diagnosed with a pontine lesion.

8.   A 55-year-old man was diagnosed with a medial longitudinal fasciculus lesion.

Themes: Agnosias

Options for questions: 9–11

A   Agraphognosia
B   Anosognosia
C   Astereognosia

D   Autopagnosia
E   Simultagnosia
F   Prosopagnosia

For each of the following descriptions, select the single most appropriate agnosia. Each option may be used once, more than once or not at all.

9.   A 38-year-old man had a stroke recently. Since then he has been unable to name or recognise the parts of his body.

10. A 71-year-old woman had a stroke recently. Since then she had demonstrated a distinct lack of awareness of her condition.

11. A 75-year- old man had a stroke recently. Since then he has been unable to recognise coins or other objects if they were placed in his hands while his eyes closed.

Theme: Levels of consciousness

Options for questions: 12–15

A   Clouding of consciousness
B   Coma
C   Oneiroid state
D   Semi-coma

E   Somnolence
F   Stupor
G   Torpor
H   Twilight state

For each of the following descriptions, select the single most appropriate consciousness state. Each option may be used once, more than once or not at all.

12. A 51-year-old man had developed a stroke recently. On examination, you noticed a variable level of consciousness that was characterised by acute onset and variable duration, and associated with emotional outbursts.

13. A 21-year-old man had a bad trip on LSD (lysergic acid diethylamide). He was brought to the accident and emergency department by his parents. On examination, he was observed to be irritable, excitable, talking to fairies and seeing elephants flying around the hospital.

14. A 79-year-old woman had developed a stroke recently. She responded to verbal commands and moved her limbs on painful stimuli and loud sounds.

15. A 31-year-old man had sustained a mild head injury recently. On examination, he was drowsy and kept falling asleep.

Theme: Side effects

Options for questions: 16–18

A	Benzhexol	D	Diuretics
B	Cycloserine	E	L-Dopa
C	Digitalis	F	Methyl dopa

For each of the following side-effect profiles, select the single most appropriate medication that is known to cause these side effects. Each option may be used once, more than once or not at all.

16. Acute organic syndrome, depression and psychotic symptoms

17. Confusion, agitation and visual hallucinations

18. Weakness, apathy and depression

GENETICS

Theme: Genetic disorders

Options for questions: 19–22

A	Chromosome 11	F	Rett's syndrome
B	Hurler's disease	G	Sturge–Weber syndrome
C	Klinefelter's syndrome	H	Tay–Sachs disease
D	Myotonic dystrophy	I	VCSF
E	Phenylketonuria	J	Xq27

For each of the following signs/symptoms, select the single most appropriate diagnosis. Each option may be used once, more than once or not at all.

19. Corneal clouding

20. Cardiotocography

21. Gaze

22. Macular cherry-red spot

Theme: Genomes

Options for questions: 23–25

A	Geonomics	E	Replication
B	Genotype	F	Ribosome
C	Metabolone	G	Splicing
D	Phenotype	H	Transcriptome

For each of the following descriptions, select the single most appropriate option. Each option may be used once, more than once or not at all.

23. A study of the sum total of DNA within an organism

24. The science of differences in DNA sequences

25. The science of differences in observable traits

ADVANCED PSYCHOLOGICAL PROCESSES AND TREATMENTS: PERSONALITY DISORDERS

Theme: Classification of personality disorders

Options for questions: 26–28

A   Antisocial personality disorder
B   Avoidant personality disorder
C   Borderline personality disorder
D   Dependent personality disorder
E   Histrionic personality disorder
F   Narcissistic personality disorder
G   Obsessive–compulsive personality disorder
H   Paranoid personality disorder
I   Schizoid personality disorder
J   Schizotypal personality disorder

For each of the following clusters, select the most appropriate personality disorder/disorders as per the instruction. Each option may be used once, more than once or not at all.

26. Cluster A (select THREE options)

27. Cluster B (select THREE options)

28. Cluster C (select TWO options)

EPIDEMIOLOGY

Theme: Epidemiological studies

Options for questions: 29–31

A   Aetiology and ethnicity of schizophrenia and other psychoses study
B   Determinants of outcome of severe mental disorders study
C   European study of the epidemiology of mental disorders survey
D   IPSS (International Pilot Study of Schizophrenia) study
E   Netherlands mental health survey and incidence study
F   PRiSM psychosis study
G   Sterling county study
H   UK700 study

For each of the following descriptions, select the single most appropriate epidemiological study that best describes it. Each option may be used once, more than once or not at all.

29. This study tried to answer questions: Can gains of experimental studies that have demonstrated benefits arising from treatment by community mental health teams be translated to routine settings? If so, are the benefits diluted in ordinary clinical practice? What were the costs?

30. This study looked at the benefits of reducing case-load size for teams looking after people with enduring mental illness.

31. This study was a 40-year perspective on the epidemiology of psychotic disorder in adult populations in Atlantic Canada.

ADVANCED PSYCHOLOGICAL PROCESSES

Theme: Family therapy

Options for questions: 32–34

A	Corrective emotional experience	E	Strategic systemic therapy
B	Family systems approach	F	Structural model
C	Milan's systemic approach	G	Dynamic model
D	Paradoxical therapy		

For each of the following therapists, select the single most appropriate family model that is associated with them. Each option may be used once, more than once or not at all.

32. Bateson

33. Minuchin

34. Palazzoli

Theme: Group therapy

Options for questions: 35–37

A	Alexander	D	Minuchin
B	Bion	E	Moreno
C	Foulkes	F	Yalom

For each of the following theories of group therapy, select the single most appropriate proponent. Each option may be used once, more than once or not at all.

35. Curative factors that act within a group therapy setting

36. Three basic states of group dynamics: dependence, fight/flight and pairing

37. Therapeutic dramatisation of emotional problems in the group

Theme: Ego defence mechanism and their actions

Options for questions: 38–40

A	Denial	F	Rationalisation
B	Displacement	G	Reaction formation
C	Identification	H	Regression
D	Isolation	I	Repression
E	Projection		

For each of the following examples, select the single most appropriate ego defence mechanism. Each option may be used once, more than once or not at all.

38. Being considerate or polite to someone you dislike, even going out of the way to be nice to them.

39. 'I hate you' gets converted to 'you hate me'.

40. Talking about a traumatic experience without showing much emotion.

Answers: EMIs

1. F Plasma aldosterone and renin measurement

Hyperaldosteronism is excess production of aldosterone. Of cases 50% are due to unilateral adrenocortical adenomas. The test used to diagnose the condition is plasma aldosterone and renin measurement.

2. G Parathyroid hormone

Hypoparathyroidism is cause by decreased secretion of parathyroid hormone. It could be because of gland failure such as removal of a gland in neck surgery. Features of hypocalcaemia are present such as depression, tetany, perioral paraesthesia and carpopedal spasm.

3. H Short ACTH stimulation test

Addison's disease is caused by adrenal insufficiency. Clinicians can diagnose anorexia nervosa or viral infection in error. Eighty per cent of cases in the UK are autoimmune, characterised by signs of hyperpigmentation, vitiligo and postural hypotension. The short adrenocorticotropic hormone (ACTH) stimulation test is specific to diagnose the condition. In Addison's disease, ACTH levels are > 300 ng/L.

4. I Thyroid antibodies

Graves' disease is commonly seen in patients aged between 30 and 50 years. The male:female ratio is 9:1. Diffuse thyroid enlargement is seen. It is also associated with normochromic/normocytic anaemia, increased erythrocyte sedimentation rate, increased calcium levels, increased liver function tests, pernicious anaemia and type 1 diabetes mellitus. Patients are mostly hyperthyroid. Thyroid-stimulating hormone receptor antibodies are seen.

5. J Thyroid-stimulating hormone

If a clinician suspects hypothyroidism in a patient, the best test that should be asked for is T_4 levels and thyroid-stimulating hormone (TSH) measures. T_3 does not add extra information. If T_4 is low and level of TSH is high then primary hypothyroidism is confirmed. If T_4 is normal and TSH is high then subclinical hypothyroidism is confirmed. Hypothyroidism can present with symptoms such as tiredness, lethargy, weight gain, cold intolerance, hoarseness of voice, depression and poor cognition.

6. D Skew deviation

Table 8.1 Skew deviation		
Clinical finding	**Lesion**	**Disease/aetiology**
Skew deviation	Brain-stem lesion	Brain-stem infarction, multiple sclerosis, tumour

---

7. B Lateral gaze palsy

Table 8.2 Lateral gaze palsy

Clinical finding	Lesion	Disease/aetiology
Lateral gaze palsy	Frontal, parietal or pontine lesion	Brain-stem infarction, multiple sclerosis, tumour

---

8. A Internuclear ophthalmoplegia

Table 8.3 Ophthalmoplegia

Clinical finding	Lesion	Disease/aetiology
Skew deviation	Brain-stem lesion	Brainstem infarction, multiple sclerosis, tumours
Single nerve palsy (III, IV or VI)	Nuclear or course of the nerve	Diabetes mellitus, aneurysm, tumours, trauma
Lateral gaze palsy	Frontal, parietal or pontine lesion	Brain-stem infarction, multiple sclerosis, tumours
Vertical gaze palsy	Upper brain-stem lesion	Brain-stem infarction, multiple sclerosis, tumours
Internuclear ophthalmoplegia	Medial longitudinal fasciculus	Multiple sclerosis
Supranuclear palsy		Degenerative condition

---

9. D Autopagnosia

Unable to name or recognise the part of the body (see **Table 8.4**).

---

10. B Anosognosia

Unawareness of the disease such as paraplegia (see **Table 8.4**).

11. C Astereognosia

Table 8.4 Agnosias
Agraphognosia or agraphaesthesia: inability to identify the letters traced on a palm with a closed eye
Anosognosia: unawareness of disease such as paraplegia
Autotopagnosia: unable to name or recognise part of the body
Astereognosia: unable to recognise the object on palpation
Simultoagnosia: unable to recognise the overall meaning of an object but the individual details are recognised
Prosopagnosia: inability to recognise the face

12. C Oneiroid state

Well-defined interruption of the continuity of consciousness which is characterised by acute onset and variable duration, and is associated with emotional outbursts (see **Table 8.5**).

13. H Twilight state

Prolonged oneiroid state with hallucinations (see **Table 8.5**).

14. F Stupor

The person is responding verbally and by motor activities to pain and loud sounds (see **Table 8.5**).

15. G Torpor

The patient is drowsy and easily falls asleep (see **Table 8.5**).

Table 8.5 Levels of consciousness
Clouding of consciousness: drowsiness and no reaction to stimuli
Coma: do response and reflexes
Oneiroid state: well-defined interruption of the continuity of consciousness which is characterised by acute onset and variable duration, and is associated with emotional outbursts
Semi coma: able to withdraw from the source of pain but there is no spontaneous motor activity
Somnolence: can be awoken, able to speak but keeps on falling asleep
Stupor: person is responding verbally and by motor activities to pain and loud sounds
Torpor: patient is drowsy and easily falls asleep
Twilight state: prolonged oneiroid state with hallucinations

16. E L-Dopa

Anti-parkinson medication such as L-dopa can give rise to an acute organic syndrome, depression and psychotic symptoms.

17. A Benzhexol

Anticholinergic drugs such as procyclidine, benztropine and benzhexol are associated with disorientation, agitation and visual hallucinations.

18. F Methyl dopa

Antihypertensive medication such as methyl dopa is associated with tiredness, weakness and depression.

Digitalis use can give rise to disorientation and mood disturbances.

Diuretics use is associated with weakness and depression due to electrolyte disturbances.

19. B Hurler's disease

Hurler's disease, which is also called gargoylism, is an autosomal recessive disorder. It is an accumulation of mucopolysaccharidoses which affect the brain as well. There is an increase in head size, hepatosplenomegaly, thick long bones, corneal clouding and kyphosis.

20. D Myotonic dystrophy

In myotonic dystrophy, there is a repeat of cardiotocography, in fragile X sydrome there is a repeat of CGG, and in Huntington's disease there is a repeat of CAG.

21. F Rett's syndrome

This is inherited as X-linked dominant condition. It is a pervasive neurodevelopmental disorder with a prevalence of 1:10,000–1:12,000 in girls. There is pervasive growth failure, communication dysfunction, and stereotypical movements. Approximately 99.5% of cases are a single occurrence in a family. Gene mutation occurs in the *MECP2* gene. Gaze is the patient's most important way of interacting as other ways of communication are quite compromised. It is the inability to perform motor functions that is the most disabling feature of Rett's syndrome, interfering with every body movement, including eye gaze and speech, although gaze is the most important way of interacting with the environment and patients show their interest by eye pointing. Developmental deviations are apparent by 15 months of age in 50%, by 18 months in 80% and by 2 years in 100%.

22. H Tay–Sachs disease

This is autosomal recessive. Tay–Sachs disease is a defect of hexosaminidase A leading to ganglioside GM2 accumulation in grey matter. An early sign is exaggerated startle which is also called hyperacusis. Macular cherry-red spot is characteristic.

23. A Genomics

This is the study of entire genomes. Genomics has been made possible by the technologies of high-throughput DNA sequencing and competition. Genetics and genetic epidemiology are a direct beneficiary of genomics.

24. B Genotype

As a science, genetics is an attempt to correlate differences in DNA sequences (genotype) with differences in observable traits (phenotype).

25. D Phenotype

It is important to differentiate between the terms 'genotype' and 'phenotype'. Genotype is a sequence of DNA material that is inherited by an organism from its parents, whereas phenotype is the observable physical and behavioural features of the organism. All the proteins expressed in an organism are proteomes and metabolone applies to enzymes it is metabolone.

26. H, I, J Paranoid personality disorder. Schizoid personality disorder. Schizotypal personality disorder

Cluster A includes three main personality disorders in which odd and unusual behaviour is common. These disorders include paranoid, schizoid and schizotypal disorders.

27. A, C, E Antisocial personality disorder. Borderline personality disorder. Histrionic personality disorder

Cluster B includes four main personality disorders in which emotional disturbance, and unpredictable and dramatic behaviour are common. These disorders include antisocial, borderline, histrionic and narcissistic personality disorder.

28. B, D Avoidant personality disorder. Dependent personality disorder

Cluster C includes a group of personality disorders in which anxiety and fear are significant. The three main disorders included in this cluster are avoidant, dependent and obsessive–compulsive personality disorder.

29. F PRiSM psychosis study

The PRiSM psychosis study was a study in the mid-1990s into community treatment of psychiatric patients in London, mainly in two catchment areas: Nunhead and Norwood under the South London and Maudsley Hospital. It concluded that community treatment of patients reduced cost of and need for inpatient admissions, increased satisfaction among patients and, overall, was similar to hospital-based treatment in most of the outcomes. However, there was no additional benefit in reducing symptom burden, family burden or social interaction.

30. H UK 700 study

This study looked at the benefits of reducing case load size for teams looking after people with enduring mental illness.

31. G Sterling county study

The Sterling county study was a 40-year perspective on epidemiology of psychotic disorder in adult populations in Atlantic Canada.

32. D Paradoxical therapy

In Bateson's paradoxical therapy the therapist makes the patient intentionally engage in unwanted behaviours called the paradoxical injunction.

33. F Structural model

Minuchin's structural model views family as a structure built of interpersonal relationships.

34. C Milan systematic approach

The Milan systemic approach by Palazzoli emphasises circular and reflexive questioning.

Bowen's model of the family systems approach emphasises one's ability to retain own's individual self in the face of familial tension. Strategic systemic therapy, according to Haley, states that symptoms are maintained by behaviours that seek to suppress them in the first place.

35. F Yalom

Curative factors that act in a group setting were developed by Yalom. In total, he described 11 factors. These factors include universality, altruism and instillation of hope, guidance, imparting information, developing social skills, interpersonal learning, cohesion, catharsis, existential factors, imitative behaviour and corrective recapitulation of family and origin issues.

36. B Bion

According to Bion, whenever a group gets derailed from its task, it deteriorates into one of three basic states: dependency, pairing or fight–flight.

37. E Moreno

Jacob Moreno founded psychodrama in which therapeutic dramatisation of emotional problems is the main principle employed.

Foulkes was regarded as one of the founders of group therapy and described a network of all individual mental processes; the psychological medium in which they meet, communicate and interact can be called the matrix, which is the hypothetical web of communication and relationship in a given group.

38. G Reaction formation

This is being considerate or polite to someone you dislike, even going out of the way to be nice to them. During reaction formation the person consciously feels or thinks the opposite of what the 'unconscious' believes. It is an intermediate defence mechanism according to Vaillant's hierarchy of defences.

39. E Projection

'I hate you' gets converted to 'you hate me'. Projection is displacing one's own unacceptable feelings/characteristics onto someone else. This happens through reversal of subject/object. It is an immature defence mechanism according to Vaillant's hierarchy of defences.

40. D Isolation

This involves talking about a traumatic experience without showing much emotion or even giggling about it. Isolation refers to separating contradictory thoughts/feelings into 'logic-tight' compartments.

Chapter 9

Test questions: 4

Questions: EMIs

Theme: Expression of genes

Options for questions: 1–4

A   Autosomal aneuploidy
B   Fragmented penetrance
C   Genetic amplification
D   Genetic anticipation
E   Genetic imprinting

F   Locus heterogeneity
G   Pleiotropy
H   Premutation
I   Reciprocal translocation

For each of the following descriptions, select the single most appropriate answer. Each option may be used once, more than once or not at all.

1.   This is represented by a diagnosis of fragile X syndrome in the son of a 30-year-old woman of average intelligence. Her husband's family has no history of fragile X syndrome, but her maternal uncle is suspected to have the same condition.

2.   This is represented by patients with Prader–Willi and Angelman's syndromes.

3.   Huntington's disease is an example of this type of gene expression.

4.   Down's syndrome is an example of this type of gene expression.

GENETICS

Theme: Genetic linkage and mutation

Options for questions: 5–9

A	Frame shift mutation	F	Pedigree-based linkage
B	Gene duplication or chromosomal duplication	G	Sequence nutation
		H	Silent mutation
C	Intronic mutation	I	Single nucleotide polymorphism and microsatellites
D	Missense mutation		
E	Nonsense mutation	J	Single nucleotide polymorphisms

For each of the following descriptions, select the single most appropriate linkage and mutation that best describe it. Each option may be used once, more than once or not at all.

5. Genetic markers are useful to identify disease genes.

6. It had been useful in identifying many genes associated with intellectual disability and dementia.

7. Changes in a single base-pair (say from C to T) in the coding sequence of a gene cause an alteration of the function of the protein.

8. Changes in a single base-pair (say from C to T) in the coding sequence of a gene result in premature termination of the protein.

9. Deletions or insertions (of any size) not affecting a multiple of three bases produce abnormal protein.

Theme: Behavioural genetics

Options for questions: 10–13

A	Concordance rates	F	Independent assortment
B	Dependent assortment	G	Intraclass correlational coefficient
C	Dichotomous characteristics	H	Logarithm of odds score
D	Double back-cross mating	I	Morbid risk
E	Heritability	J	Recombination fraction

For each of the following statements, select the single most appropriate option. Each option may be used once, more than once or not at all.

10. How is twins similarity for continuous traits expressed?

11. How is twins similarity for dichotomous characteristics expressed?

12. On what is Mendel's law of inheritance based?

13. As what is transmission of phenotypic traits that occurs when genes for these traits are located far apart on the same or different chromosome known?

ADVANCED PSYCHOLOGICAL PROCESSES AND TREATMENTS: PERSONALITY DISORDERS

Theme: Persons associated with personality disorders

Options for questions: 14–16

A	Cleckley	F	Jung
B	Eysenck	G	Kraepelin
C	Freud	H	Klein
D	Henderson	I	Pinel
E	Hippocrates	J	Schneider

For each of the following statements on personality disorder, select the single most appropriate person involved with that personality disorder. Each option may be used once, more than once or not at all.

14. Who first described the concept of sociopathy?

15. Who first described psychopathic personality in 1906?

16. Who divided psychopathic states into aggressive, inadequate and creative?

EPIDEMIOLOGY

Theme: Epidemiological studies

Options for questions: 17–18

A	Aetiology and ethnicity of schizophrenia and other psychoses study	D	International paediatric stroke study
B	Determinants of outcome of severe mental disorders study	E	Netherlands mental health survey and incidence study
C	European study of the epidemiology of mental disorders (ESEMED) survey	F	Prism psychosis study
		G	Sterling county study
		H	UK 700 study

For each of the following descriptions/outcomes, select the single most appropriate epidemiological study. Each option may be used once, more than once or not at all.

17. The aim of the study was to investigate the prevalence and correlates of suicidal ideas and attempts in the general population of Europe.

18. This study looked at a large first presentation sample of psychotic disorders. It looked at aetiology and ethnicity in these groups.

GENETICS

Theme: Patterns of inheritance

Options for questions: 19–23

A	Autosomal dominant	F	Transcription
B	Autosomal recessive	G	Translation
C	Oligogenic	H	X-linked recessive
D	Polygenic	I	X-linked dominant
E	Polymorphism	J	Y linked

For each of the following statements, select the single most appropriate correct term described with regard to inheritance. Each option may be used once, more than once or not at all.

19. Both parents are usually unaffected heterozygotes.

20. Parents are an affected homozygote and an unaffected heterozygote.

21. Risk increased through a combination of susceptibility loci.

22. Traits are inherited only from the father.

23. Mother is a carrier and father is unaffected.

Theme: Complications to pedigree patterns

Options for questions: 24–28

A	Autosomal dominant	F	Non-penetrance
B	Dynamic mutation	G	Oligogenic
C	Genomic imprinting	H	Polygenic
D	Locus heterogeneity	I	X-linked recessive
E	Mitochondrial inheritance	J	Y linked

For each of the following statements, select the single most appropriate term that best describes it. Each option may be used once, more than once or not at all.

24. Mutations in several different genes result in the same phenotype.

25. Despite dominant inheritance pattern, a generation is skipped.

26. Mitochondrial mutations result in maternal patterns of transmission.

27. Differential expression of genes depends on whether the chromosome is derived maternally or paternally.

28. DNA mutation occurs during transmission from one generation to the next.

Theme: Genetic studies

Options for questions: 29–31

A Adoptee's family strategy	F Family study method
B Adoption strategy	G Genomic imprinting
C Cross-fostering design	H Monozygotic twins
D Dynamic mutation	I Pairwise concordance rate (CR)
E Family history method	J Probandwise CR

For each of the following statements, select the single most appropriate genetic study described. Each option may be used once, more than once or not at all.

29. Diagnoses are obtained by interviewing each family member.

30. Twin study designs examine the concordance between affected and unaffected.

31. Information is gathered by interviewing the proband.

Theme: Terms used in genetics

Options for questions: 32–36

A Autosomal dominant	G Polymorphism
B Heterozygous	H Transcription
C Homozygous	I Translation
D Genotype	J X-linked recessive
E Oligogenic	K Y linked
F Phenotype	

For each of the following, select the single most appropriate term that describes it. Each option may be used once, more than once or not at all.

32. The physically observable characteristics

33. DNA variants satisfactorily common in the general population

34. Combination of alleles on the loci of a chromosome

35. Two alleles the same in an individual

36. Two alleles different in an individual

Answers: EMIs

1. H Premutation

This is described as a situation in which someone harbours the trinucleotide expansion but it is not long enough for it to produce the disease in the probands. However, premutation will produce further expansion of the loci during cell divisions if children of the affected person inherit the genes. They will then express the mutation and develop the disease, unlike their parents.

2. E Genomic imprinting

The expression of disease phenotype depends on the allele of maternal or paternal lineage and it is called genomic imprinting. Both Prader–Willi and Angelman's syndromes are associated with genomic imprinting on chromosome 15q-11–q13. However, about 70% of the former patients have deletion in the paternally derived chromosome and about 95% of the latter patients have a deletion in the maternally derived chromosome.

3. D Genetic anticipation

The phenomenon in which the phenotype expression of a mutation occurs earlier and earlier in successive generations is called genetic anticipation. This is also observed in some of the trinucleotide repeat diseases.

4. A Autosomal aneuploidy

In this form of gene expression, the diseases are not inherited from parents but show a correlation with the mother's mother's age. This is probably due to the fact that an ageing ovum is more prone to cell division errors.

Pleiotropy means that a single gene defect leads to multiple defects in a variety of organs, e.g. Marfan's syndrome, which is due to an autosomal dominant mutation. When mutations in multiple genes in different chromosomes cause a single disorder or trait, it is called locus heterogeneity. In reciprocal translocation, an exchange of genetic material takes place between two chromosomes. People carrying reciprocal translocation may not be clinically affected, because they do not possess the full complement of essential genetic material. However, their children may inherit partial trisomy or partial monosomy of the exchanged genetic material.

5. I Single nucleotide polymorphism and microsatellites

Availability of genetic markers assists in molecular mapping. There are additional small repeated DNA sequences, most commonly cytosine and adenine, which differ in length among different individuals. One of them is short tandem repeats or microsatellites, which occur almost every 50 kilobases and have no phenotypic significance. Other, more complex sequence polymorphisms are single nucleotide polymorphisms (SNPs), which along with microsatellites are most useful for identifying disease genes. A point mutation occurring in non-coding DNA regions, i.e. SNPs, do not have any effect on the phenotype but are very useful genetic markers for identification of an individual and in determining of paternity.

6. F Pedigree-based linkage

This works well when a disease follows simple mendelian laws of segregation. Pedigree-based linkage (PBL) has helped in identifying many genes involved in intellectual disability and dementia.

However, if genetic effect-size attributable to a single locus is small, PBL will require an impractically large number of families, and in that case a direct test of association between genetic marker and the disease gene is much more reliable. Gene mutation is a type of mutation in which a portion of a genetic material (DNA or a chromosome-containing gene) is duplicated or replicated, generating multiple copies of that portion

7. D Missense mutation

Permanent changes in the sequences of genomic DNA are known as mutations. Changes in a single base-pair (say from C to T) in the coding sequence of a gene, causing an alteration of the function of the protein s are called missense mutations

8. E Nonsense mutation

Changes in a single base pair, say from C to T, in the coding sequence of a gene result in premature termination of the protein.

9. A Frame-shift mutation

Deletions or insertions (of any size) not affecting a multiple of three bases change the way that a genetic message is translated, and the protein produced could be shorter or longer than it should be and most probably useless. When the DNA mutation occurs either in a non-coding region, i.e. outside a gene, or within an intron or an exon in a way that it does not alter the final amino acid sequence of the protein, it is called a silent mutation.

10. G Intraclass correlational coefficient

Twin similarity for continuous traits such as height, weight is expressed as an intra class correlational coefficient

11. A Concordance rates

Twin similarity for dichotomous characteristics is expressed as a concordance rate. A probandwise concordance rate is the number of affected twins divided by the total number of co-twins. A pairwise concordance rate is the number of twin pairs having the disorder divided by the total number of twin pairs.

12. C Dichotomous characteristics

Mendel's laws of inheritance are based on dichotomous characteristics that are may or may not be affected by a disorder. These can also be applied for continuous characteristics such as weight, height and blood pressure.

13. F Independent assortment

Transmission of phenotypic traits, which occurs when genes for these traits are located far apart on the same or a different chromosome is known as independent assortment. Dependent assortment occurs when the loci are close together. However, if the loci are very close to each other, recombination or crossing over rarely occurs and the recombination fraction is zero. The relative influence of genetic factors on a phenotype is called heritability.

The most appropriate method to correct for age in analysis of genetic disorders is morbid risk. Double back-cross mating is the mating between a double heterozygote and a homozygote.

14. A Cleckley

In 1955, Cleckley identified sociopathy and described a sociopath as someone who is unreliable and untruthful, lacks remorse and is antisocial.

15. G Kraepelin

Emil Kraepelin described psychopathic personality, including excitable, unstable and quarrelsome subtypes.

16. D Henderson

Psychopathic state is subdivided into three subtypes such as aggressive, inadequate and creative. This concept was described by Henderson.

17. C European study of the epidemiology of mental disorders (ESEMED) survey

The aim of the study was to investigate the prevalence and correlates of suicidal ideas and attempts in the general population of Europe.

18. A Aetiology and ethnicity of schizophrenia and other psychoses study

This study looked at a large first presentation sample of psychotic disorders. They looked at aetiology and ethnicity in these groups.

19. B Autosomal recessive

Both parents are usually unaffected heterozygotes.

20. A Autosomal dominant

Parents are an affected homozygote and an unaffected heterozygote.

21. D Polygenic

Risk is increased through a combination of susceptibility loci.

22. J Y-linked

Traits inherited only from the father are Y-linked traits.

23. H X-linked recessive

The mother is a carrier of the gene and the father is unaffected.

Mendelian inheritance patterns are as follows:

- Autosomal dominant in which the parents are an affected homozygote and an unaffected heterozygote

- Autosomal recessive in which both parents are usually unaffected heterozygotes
- X-linked recessive in which the mother is an unaffected heterozygote or carrier and the father unaffected
- X-linked dominant in which the mother is affected and the father unaffected with a 1:1 ratio of affected to unaffected offspring or the father is affected but the mother is unaffected, resulting in daughters who are completely affected but not the sons
- Y-linked in which traits are inherited only from the father

Non-mendelian patterns of inheritance are:

- Oligogenic in which there are susceptibility genes at relatively few loci which increase the risk but individually are not enough to have an influence
- Polygenic in which the risk increased through a combination of susceptibility loci

Polymorphism is an allelic variation. Transcription and translation are cell processes.

24. D Locus heterogeneity

Mutations in several different genes result in the same phenotype.

25. F Non-penetrance

Despite dominant inheritance pattern, a generation is skipped.

26. E Mitochondrial inheritance

Mitochondrial mutations result in maternal patterns of transmission.

27. C Genomic imprinting

This is differential expression of genes depending on whether the chromosome is derived maternally or paternally.

28. B Dynamic mutation

DNA mutation occurs during transmission from one generation to the next.

The following are complications to pedigree patterns:

- Dynamic mutation in which DNA mutation occurs during transmission from generation to the next
- Genomic imprinting in which there is differential expression of genes depending on whether the chromosome is derived maternally or paternally
- Locus heterogeneity in which mutations in several different genes result in the same phenotype
- Mitochondrial inheritance: mitochondrial mutations result in maternal patterns of transmission
- Non-penetrance in which, despite a dominant inheritance pattern, a generation is skipped

Mendelian inheritance patterns are:

- Autosomal dominant
- Autosomal recessive
- X-linked recessive
- X-linked dominant
- Y-linked

Non-mendelian patterns of inheritance are:

- Oligogenic
- Polygenic

29. F Family study method

Diagnoses obtained by interviewing each family member.

30. H Monozygotic twins

Twin study designs examine the concordance between affected and unaffected twins.

31. E Family history method

Information is gathered interviewing the proband.

In genetic epidemiology studies, the three main study designs are adoption, family and twin studies.

Examples are:

- Adoption studies: examples of this are adoptee strategy and adoption family strategy.
- Family studies: family history method is where information is gathered interviewing the proband or a relative about the diagnoses of the other family members. Family study method is where diagnoses are obtained by interviewing each family member.
- Twin studies look at monozygotic and dizygotic twin pairs. Pairwise and probandwise concordance rates are used to calculate the concordance.

Genomic imprinting and dynamic mutation are complications of pedigree patterns.

32. F Phenotype

This is the physically observable characteristics.

33. G Polymorphism

It refers to DNA variants that are satisfactorily common in the general population (minimum 1%).

34. D Genotype

The combination of alleles on the loci of a chromosome is the genotype.

35. C Homozygous

It happens when the two alleles are the same in an individual.

36. B Heterozygous

This happens where the two alleles are different in an individual.

The phenotype is the term used when looking at the physically observable characteristics of an organism. Autosomal dominant, oligogenic, X-linked recessive and Y-linked are patterns of inheritance.

Chapter 10

Mock examination

Questions: EMIs

EXTENDED MATCHING ITEMS

Theme: Behaviour modification techniques

Options for questions: 1–4

A   Extinction
B   Modelling
C   Negative reinforcement
D   Premack's principle
E   Punishment
F   Schedules of reinforcement
G   Shaping
H   Social rewards
I   Stimulus control
J   Time out
K   Token system

For each of the following cases, select the single most appropriate behavioural technique that can be used. Each option may be used once, more than once or not at all.

1. A 37-year-old man kept playing on the slot machines. He continued to play, hoping to have a big win because once in a while he had a small one.

2. A 5-year-old girl had gradually been oriented to her gender of being a girl by her parents who had introduced her to pink clothes and playing with dolls.

3. A 20-year-old male college student found revision boring and difficult. His father, after observing what he liked, promised him a treat of buying him music DVDs of his choice so he continued revising his studies.

4. A 16-year-old girl with a learning disability found the loud noise of the garbage removal truck every Friday during her morning walk intolerable. She responded with head banging or hitting out at others. Her carers had changed her routine to remain inside on Friday morning by engaging in art work and she went out only later in the day.

Theme: Genetic epidemiology

Options for questions 5–9

A	Biochemical genetics	E	Molecular genetics
B	Developmental genetics	F	Population genetics
C	Evolutionary genetics	G	Psychiatric genetics
D	Genetic demography	H	Quantitative genetics

For each of the following statements, select the single most appropriate terminology that best describes it. Each option may be used once, more than once or not at all.

5. It is a study of how the expression of normal genes controls growth and other maturational processes.

6. It is a study of chemical reactions by which genetic determinants are replicated and produce their effects.

7. It is a study of the structure and functions of genes at a molecular level.

8. It deals with the mathematical properties of genetic transmission in families and populations.

9. It is a study of changes in gene frequency across generations.

Theme: Brain structures

Options for questions: 10–14

A	Amygdala	G	Globus pallidus
B	Brain stem	H	Hippocampus
C	Caudate nucleus	I	Mammillary bodies
D	Cerebellum	J	Medial geniculate body
E	Cerebral cortex	K	Premotor cortex
F	Corpus callosum	L	Putamen

For each of the following components, select the most appropriate brain structure(s) that is associated with it as per further instructions. Each option may be used once, more than once or not at all.

10. Mossy fibres (select ONE option)

11. Largest white matter structure (select ONE option)

12. Limbic system (select THREE options)

13. Lenticular nucleus (select TWO options)

14. Thalamus (select ONE option)

Theme: Contribution to development of psychological theories

Options for questions: 15–17

A   Albert Ellis
B   Anna Freud
C   Bandura
D   Cohen
E   Erik Erikson
F   Gould
G   Hobbes
H   Kelly
I   Meddis

For each of the following psychological theories, select the single most appropriate person involved with it. Each option may be used once, more than once or not at all.

15. Personal construct theory

16. Social learning theory

17. Theory of hedonism

Theme: Study designs for clinical research

Options for questions: 18–21

A   Case–control study
B   Cohort study
C   Cluster randomised trial
D   Cross-over randomised trial
E   Cross-sectional survey
F   Ecological study
G   Economical analysis
H   Parallel randomised trial
I   Retrospective cohort study
J   Open-label randomised controlled trial
K   Prospective cohort
L   Qualitative study

For each of the following study questions, select the single most appropriate study design. Each option may be used once, more than once or not at all.

18. To find an association between delivery complications and development of psychosis with minimum attrition bias.

19. To find an association between use of Depakote in pregnancy and development of spina bifida in the offspring.

20. To find out the cut-off point in a new rating scale using the ICD-10 criteria.

21. To elicit the patient's view about treatment and reason of disengagement.

Theme: Topographical model of the mind

Options for questions: 22–23

A   Desires are viewed as weak and unacceptable, therefore extinguished
B   Evident via parapraxes (freudian slips) and dreams
C   Governed by the pleasure principle
D   Contents communicated via speech and behaviour

E   Maintains the 'repressive barrier' to censor unacceptable wishes and desires (not the repressed contents)
F   Receives and processes information from outside world
G   Repressed memories communicated directly through speech
H   Shift of cathexis not possible

For each of the following areas of mind according to topographical model of mind, select the most appropriate activities as per instructions. Each option may be used once, more than once or not at all.

22. Unconscious (select TWO options)

23. Preconscious (select ONE option)

Theme: Genetic disorders

Options for questions: 24–25

A   Chromosome 11 deletion
B   Hurler's syndrome
C   Klinefelter's syndrome
D   Myotonic dystrophy
E   Phenylketonuria

F   Rett's syndrome
G   Sturge–Weber syndrome
H   Tay-Sachs disease
I   Velocardiofacial syndrome
J   XYY syndrome

For each of the following signs/symptoms, select the single most appropriate diagnosis. Each option may be used once, more than once or not at all.

24. Mousy odour, fits, fair hair, blue eyes, eczema and cerebral palsy

25. Schneider's first rank symptoms, persecutory delusions, negative symptoms

Theme: Contributions to psychological theories and therapies

Options for questions: 26–28

A   Albert Ellis
B   Bem
C   Cohen
D   Eisenberg
E   Kohlberg

F   Lorenz
G   Main
H   Oswalds
I   Piaget

For each of the following theories/therapies, select the single most appropriate contributor. Each option may be used once, more than once or not at all.

26. Rational–emotive behaviour therapy

27. Stages of moral development

28. Theory of moral development

Theme: Psychological management of mental disorders

Options for questions: 29–32

A   Brief psychodynamic psychotherapy
B   Cognitive–analytical therapy
C   Cognitive–behaviour therapy
D   Dialectical behaviour therapy

E   Eye movement desensitisation and reprocessing
F   Flooding
G   Interpersonal therapy
H   Systematic desensitisation

For each of the following conditions, select the single most appropriate therapy. Each option may be used once, more than once or not at all.

29. Depression

30. Emotionally unstable personality disorder–borderline type

31. Agoraphobia

32. Post-traumatic stress disorder

Theme: Genomes

Options for questions: 33–34

A   Geonomics
B   Genotype
C   Metabolon
D   Phenotype

E   Replication
F   Ribosome
G   Splicing
H   Transcription

For each of the following cases, select the single most appropriate option. Each option may be used once, more than once or not at all.

33. The sum total of RNAs expressed in an organism

34. The sum total of enzyme activities in a cell

Theme: Genetic models

Options for questions: 35–39

A   Complete penetrance
B   Epigenesis
C   Imprinting
D   Mixed model

E   Multilocus model
F   Nucleotide polymorphisms
G   Single major locus model
H   Transgenic model

For each of the following cases, select the single most appropriate genetical model. Each option may be used once, more than once or not at all.

35. It is synonymous with a mendelian model of transmission.

36. The genetic influences in this model may arise from the effects of genes of major effect vs genes of minor effect, with or without contributions from the environment.

37. Inheritance of Alzheimer's disease is understood using this model.

38. Factors are transmitted to progeny cells after cell division, but are not directly attributable to DNA sequence.

39. Huntington's disease transmission is explained by using this model.

Theme: Diagnosis of DSM-IV personality disorders

Options for questions: 40–43

A   Antisocial personality disorder
B   Avoidant personality disorder
C   Borderline personality disorder
D   Dependent personality disorder
E   Histrionic personality disorder

F   Narcissistic personality disorder
G   Obsessive–compulsive personality disorder
H   Paranoid personality disorder
I   Schizoid personality disorder
J   Schizotypal personality disorder

For each of the following cases, select the single most appropriate diagnosis. Each option may be used once, more than once or not at all.

40. The person is often envious of others or believes that others are envious of him or her.

41. The person is preoccupied with being criticised or rejected in social situations.

42. The person reads hidden demeaning or threatening meanings into benign remarks or events.

43. The person urgently seeks another relationship as a source of care and support when a close relationship ends.

Theme: Contribution to psychological theories and therapies

Options for questions: 44–47

A   Conscious and unconscious
B   Cognitive behaviourism and social learning
C   Ego psychology
D   Id, ego and super-ego
E   Individual psychology

F   Inner working models
G   Learned helplessness
H   Operant conditioning
I   Transactional analysis
J   Universal emotions

For each of the following persons, select the single most appropriate contribution they made. Each option may be used once, more than once or not at all.

44. Ainsworth

45. Carl Gustav Jung

46. Sigmund Freud

47. Skinner

Theme: Neuropsychological measures

Options for questions: 48–51

A   Behavioural assessment of the dysexecutive syndrome
B   Cambridge cognitive examination (CAMCOG)
C   Complex figure test
D   Hayling and Brixton test
E   Mini–mental state examination
F   National adult reading test
G   Test of everyday attention
H   Wechsler's abbreviated scale of intelligence
I   Wisconsin card sorting test

For each of the following descriptions, select the single most appropriate test. Each option may be used once, more than once or not at all.

48. This is used for people who sustain frontal lobe damage and includes provision of a measure of speed of initiation on a response suppression task as well as a stimulus booklet.

49. This is a widely used test of set shifting ability.

50. This is used to measure intellectual function.

51. This is widely used to test visuospatial memory.

Theme: Neuropsychology of perception

Options for questions: 52–54

A   Agnosia
B   Agraphognosia
C   Anosognosia
D   Astereognosia
E   Constructional apraxia
F   Ideational apraxia
G   Ideomotor apraxia
H   Prosopagnosia
I   Pseudoagnosia

For each of the following descriptions, select the single most appropriate neurological deficit. Each option may be used once, more than once or not at all.

52. The inability to identify numbers drawn on the palm or other parts of the body.

53. The inability to mimic a learned motor task.

54. Loss of the ability to conceptualise.

Theme: Contributions psychological theories and therapies

Options for questions: 55–57

A   Geon theory of pattern recognition
B   Gestalt therapy
C   Hierarchy of needs
D   Imprinting
E   Learned helplessness
F   Primary universal emotions
G   Psychosocial theory
H   Self-perception theory

For each of the following people, select the single most appropriate contribution that he or she made. Each option may be used once, more than once or not at all.

55. Ekman and Friesen

56. Maslow

57. Seligman

Theme: Language areas in the brain

Options for questions: 58–60

A   Angular gyrus
B   Auditory association cortex
C   Auditory cortex
D   Broca's area
E   Left cerebral hemisphere

F   Right cerebral hemisphere
G   Visual cortex
H   Wernicke's area
I   Visual association cortex

For each of the following cases, select the single most appropriate area involved in the language process. Each option may be used once, more than once or not at all.

58. Present in the inferior frontal gyrus

59. Posterior part of the superior temporal gyrus

60. BA 39

Theme: Principles of therapeutic communities

Options for questions: 61–62

A   Analytic–behavioural community
B   Concept–based community
C   Democratic analytic community
D   Democratisation
E   Mill Hill experiments

F   Northfield experiments
G   Reality confrontation
H   Rehabilitation
I   Stabilisation
J   Static conceptual community

For each of the following descriptions, select the most appropriate principles of therapeutic community according to further instructions. Each option may be used once, more than once or not at all.

61. Historically the concept of therapeutic communities stems from two different types of communities (select TWO options).

62. These are the some of the key values that held by staff with regard to treatment in a therapeutic community (select TWO options).

Theme: Principles and practice of transactional analysis

Options for questions: 63–65

A   Behavioural
B   Games
C   Good-bye letters
D   Homework
E   Humanistic
F   Interference

G   Psychoanalytic
H   Psychotherapeutic
I   Repression
J   Treatment contracts
K   Transactions

For each of the following descriptions, select the most appropriate principles/practice according to further instructions. Each option may be used once, more than once or not at all.

63. The concepts of transactional analysis and theory of personality form two types of therapies (select TWO options).

64. It is one of the distinguishing features of transactional analysis (select ONE option).

65. They are a part of the four cornerstones of transactional analysis (select TWO options).

Theme: History of personality disorders

Options for questions: 66–68

A   1
B   2
C   3
D   4
E   6
F   8

G   Melancholic
H   Moral insanity
I   Psychopathic states
J   Phlegmatic
K   Sanguine

For each of the following descriptions, select the most appropriate options according to further instructions. Each option may be used once, more than once or not at all.

66. How many temperaments did Hippocrates describe? (Select ONE option.)

67. Which of the above belong to the temperaments as described by Hippocrates? (Select TWO options.)

68. Which concept of personality from the list above was described by Prichard? (Select ONE option.)

Answers: EMIs

1. F Schedule of reinforcement

Schedules of reinforcement: these can be continuous or variable (interval or ratio). A continuous schedule is reinforcement after each behaviour. An interval variable schedule is reinforcement after a fixed time period and interval ratio is reinforcement after a certain number of behaviours.

2. G Shaping

This involves small steps towards a desired outcome when the individual cannot visualise the end-result.

3. D Premack's principle

This involves identifying reinforcers that are effective where obvious ones fail to work. It also involves observing individuals when left unattended to identify what behaviours are liked and carried out at a high frequency. This can be used as a response to target low-frequency behaviour.

4. I Stimulus control

This involves removal of a stimulus (antecedent) that leads to an unwanted behaviour rather than changing the consequences.

5. B Developmental genetics

This is a study of how genes control growth and development. It encompasses studying the growth and maturation of the study organism.

6. A Biochemical genetics

This is a study of the nature of genes and its impact on the development of the organism. It also takes into account the physical nature of the genes.

7. E Molecular genetics

This is a study of the structure and the functioning of genes at the molecular level.

8. F Population genetics

This involves studying allele distribution as part of the evolutionary process in families and populations. Population genetics also includes processes of adaptation, natural selection and mutations.

9. C Evolutionary genetics

This is the study of genetics and evolutionary processes, and the associations between them. It aims to study how genetic changes take place across long periods of time and leads to diversity in nature. Psychiatric genetics involves the study of genes to examine psychiatric disorders.

10. D Cerebellum

Along with climbing fibres, mossy fibres are the afferent fibres found in the cerebellum.

11. F Corpus callosum

This is the largest commissure in the brain. The main divisions of the corpus callosum are the rostrum, genu, body and splenium.

12. A, H, I Amygdala. Hippocampus. Mammillary bodies

There is a disagreement among the literature and academics as to which structures form a part of the limbic system. The cingulate gyrus, anterior nucleus of thalamus, septal nuclei and hypothalamus are some of the other structures included in limbic system by some authors. Some fibre bundles include cingulum, fornix, and median forebrain bundle and stria terminalis.

13. G, L Globus pallidus. Putamen

The lenticular nucleus consists of the globus pallidus and putamen.

14. J Medial geniculate body

This is a part of the auditory pathway and located in the thalamus. Similarly, the lateral geniculate body is a part of visual pathway.

15. H Kelly

Personal construct theory stressed the uniqueness of each individual and that all individuals are scientists and generate their own interpretations of the world around. Repertory grid was constructed based on Kelly's theory.

16. C Bandura

Social learning theory (SLT), described by Bandura, was later renamed social cognitive theory. According to him, reinforcements serve as informative and motivational operations rather than just as response strengtheners. SLT has been applied to aggression, moral and gender development, and personality.

17. G Hobbes

According to the theory of hedonism, seeking of pleasure and avoidance of pain determine all behaviour. This idea is central to Freud's concept of the pleasure principle. According to Hobbes, the 'real' motive behind all behaviour is pleasure, whatever we may believe.

18. A Case–control study

In this study, individuals with a particular condition or disease are selected and compared with individuals without the condition or disease. The case–control comparison is the frequency of previous exposure or attributes potentially relevant to the development of the condition under study. Such studies are relatively quick and inexpensive. They are suitable for rare diseases, but unsuitable for rare exposures. They can evaluate distant and multiple exposures.

19. K Prospective cohort

In prospective cohort studies, the population is selected before the onset of the outcome and follow-up is done for a long period.

20. E Cross-sectional survey

This measures associations of disease. It can use pre-recorded data, but it cannot distinguish between cause and effect.

21. L Qualitative study

Qualitative study measures are subjective and related to personal meanings, experiences, feelings, values and opinions.

22. B, C Governed by the pleasure principle. Evident via parapraxis (freudian slips) and dreams

The unconscious helps in maintaining the repressive barrier. Although it is not possible to access it to awareness, it still exerts influence on our actions and our conscious awareness.

23. E Maintains the 'repressive barrier' to censor unacceptable wishes and desires (not the repressed contents)

Freud described the topographical model of the mind using three areas: conscious, preconscious and unconscious. The conscious helps to think in a logical manner and holds what one is aware of. The preconscious is governed by the principle of pleasure and things stored in here can be easily brought to the conscious mind.

24. E Phenylketonuria

This is an autosomal recessive disorder, which is the third most common cause of learning disability after Down's syndrome and fragile X syndrome. It occurs in 1:14,000 livebirths. There is absence of an enzyme called phenylalanine hydroxylase, which is responsible for the conversion of phenylalanine to tyrosine. The Guthrie test, basically detects β-subtilis, the multiplication of which depends on phenylalanine. It is done 6–14 days after birth. The deficiency of phenylalanine hydroxylase can lead to severe mental retardation and this can be avoided if phenylalanine is excluded from the diet. Sufferers may present with autistic behaviour, cerebral palsy, characteristic mousy odour, fits, eczema, fair hair, blue eyes, etc.

25. C Klinefelter's syndrome

47,XXY (Klinefelter's syndrome) the male has an extra X chromosome which is maternal in 60% of cases and 15% are mosaics. The patient has small testis and is infertile with low testosterone levels. He might have gynaecomastia and may or may not have mild mental retardation. Schizophrenia is an association with Klinefelter's syndrome.

26. A Albert Ellis

Rational–emotive behaviour therapy (REBT), devised by Albert Ellis, attempts to get patients to dispute irrational and unscientific beliefs and replace them with rational beliefs. The key concept underlying REBT is that people are not disturbed by the events themselves but by their perception of such events.

27. E Kohlberg

Kohlberg's moral development is divided into three levels and six stages. The three levels are preconventional, conventional and postconventional. Each of these levels is further divided into two stages each. The preconventional level is divided into two stages: obedience/punishment orientation and self-interest orientation. The conventional stage is divided into interpersonal accord orientation and authority/social order orientation. The postconventional stage is divided into social contracts orientation and universal ethical issues orientation.

28. I Piaget

Theory of moral development was developed by Piaget who called the morality of young children heteronomous and that of older children, autonomous. According to Piaget, the shift in moral development from heteronomous to autonomous occurred at about the age of seven.

29. C Cognitive–behavioural therapy

Aaron Beck proposed cognitive–behavioural therapy initially. It addresses dysfunctional thoughts and how they impact on one's emotions and behaviours.

30. D Dialectical behaviour therapy

Marsha Linehan developed dialectical behaviour therapy (DBT). It involves individual and group work. DBT uses methods of Zen Buddhism and cognitive–behavioural therapies.

31. H Systemic desensitisation

Wolpe developed systemic desensitisation. It is based on the principle of counterconditioning whereby a completely relaxed individual is gradually introduced to an anxiety-provoking situation.

32. E Eye movement desensitisation and reprocessing

Shapiro developed eye movement desensitisation and reprocessing. Here the experience of distressing and traumatic memories or images while tracking an object in front of the line of vision using rapid eye movements yields a more positive effect and in turn a decrease in anxiety.

33. H Transcription

Genetic information is transferred from the gene to mRNA which is known as transcription.

34. C Metabolon

Genomics is the study of entire genomes. This stream of study involves examining DNA sequencing, mapping and other processes involving genes.

Genetics and genetic epidemiology are direct beneficiaries of genomics. As a science genetics is attempting to examine the impact of genotype changes on phenotypes. A transcriptome is a name given to a collection of all RNAs in an organism. These RNAs could be messenger, transfer or ribosomal RNA. All the proteins expressed in an organism is a proteome. Similarly, for enzymes it is metabolon.

35. G Single major locus model

Mendelian inheritance is also known as monogenetic inheritance. The patters of such inheritance can be examined by looking at the family tree. Mendelian trait is seen in mutations that involve a single gene locus. Some of the disorders that follow such inheritance are sickle cell anaemia, cystic fibrosis and Huntington's disease.

36. E Multilocus model

This model is based on effects of multiple loci in the causation of a disease. There may or may not be gene–environment interactions.

37. B Epigenesis

The term 'epigenesis' is often used interchangeably with epigenetic phenomenon. DNA methylation is one such epigenetic phenomenon relevant to psychiatric disorders. The *FMR1* gene, which is located on the X chromosome, is silenced by methylation in the fragile X syndrome. Other such epigenetic phenomena include gene slicing and chromosome activation. Prader–Willi syndrome and Angleman's syndrome involve imprinting, as an epigenetic phenomenon.

38. B Epigenesis

Additional factors, in addition to genetic material, following cell divisioan can be transmitted to progency cells. These cells are not directly attribuatable to DNA sequence. This process is known as epigenesis.

39. G Single major locus model

Mendelian inheritance is also known as monogenetic inheritance. The patters of such inheritance can be examined by looking at the family tree. Mendelian trait is seen in mutations that involve a single gene locus. Some of the disorders that follow such inheritance are sickle cell anaemia, cystic fibrosis and Huntington's disease.

40. F Narcissistic personality disorder

As per the DSM-IV diagnostic criteria, a patient with this disorder would suffer from a grandiose sense of self-esteem. Patients would be preoccupied with fantasies of power, appearances and success. They believe that they are special and deserve more attention than others. Such people lack empathy and are often exploitative of others. They are unwilling to recognise the needs of others. They may feel jealous of others and form beliefs that others are jealous of them. They often come across as arrogant and haughty.

41. B Avoidant personality disorder

According to the DSM-IV-TR, an individual with anxious avoidant personality disorder would avoid occupational activities involving significant interpersonal contact, is unwilling to get involved with people, resists intimate relationships, is preoccupied with being criticised, feels inadequate in him- or herself and views self as socially inept.

42. H Paranoid personality disorder

Patients with paranoid personality disorder are suspicious of others without sufficient basis. They doubt others' intentions and are reluctant to confide in other people. They are very sensitive to other people's benign remarks and read hidden, threatening or demeaning meanings into them. Patients believe that others are attacking their image or character when that is not the case. They bear grudges that remain for long periods.

43. D Dependent personality disorder

According to the DSM-IV-TR, an individual with a dependent personality disorder would have difficulty making everyday decisions, need others to assume responsibility for major areas in his or her life, struggle to express disagreement with others, struggle to initiate projects, require excessive nurturance and support from others, feel helpless when alone, and urgently require another relationship when one ends.

44. B Cognitive behaviourism and social learning

Ainsworth and Wittig, in 1969, devised the strange situation experiment. Three types of attachment behaviours were observed during the experiment type A: anxious avoidant (15%), type B: securely attached (70%) and type C: anxious resistant (15%).

Anna Freud devised adolescent analytic psychology.

Sigmund Freud's theories stimulated development of alternative theories. His daughter Anna Freud was one of the first psychologists to focus on adolescence as a key development phase. She also elaborated on many of the defence mechanisms such as regression, repression, reaction formation, isolation, undoing, projection, introjections, turning against self, reversal and sublimation.

45. A Consciousness and unconscious

According to Carl Jung, personality is present from birth. He believed that the psyche comprises consciousness and unconscious. Consciousness appears early in life through use of four basic functions, i.e. thinking, feeling, sensing and intuiting. The personal unconscious includes things that have been forgotten and also those that are in memory.

46. D Id, ego and super-ego

According to Sigmund Freud's psychoanalytic theory, personality comprises three parts: id, ego and super-ego. The id is governed by the pleasure principle and is the infantile, presocialised part of the personality. The ego is considered the 'executive' of the personality and is associated with the reality principle. It deals with planning, decision-making, rational and logical thinking, and helping postpone the satisfaction, which is demanded by the id (deferred gratification). The super-ego is considered the moral 'policeman' that threatens the ego with punishment.

47. H Operant conditioning

Skinner coined the term 'operant conditioning'. It is also known as instrumental conditioning. The learning takes place by positive and negative reinforcements. Responses that lead to positive consequences occur more frequently (positive reinforcements).

48. D Hayling and Brixton test

This is used to test for frontal lobe damage and consist of two tests, namely the Hayling and the Brixton test.

49. I Wisconsin card sorting test

This is used to test set shifting ability, which is impaired in frontal lobe damage.

50. H Wechsler abbreviated scale of intelligence

This is useful where a brief measure of intelligence is needed.

51. C Complex figure test

The Rey complex figure test has been widely used to test visuospatial memory.

52. B Agraphognosia

This is the inability to identify numbers or letters traced on the palm (or other parts of the body surface).

53. G Ideomotor apraxia

This is the inability to perform basic tasks that were earlier leant in life. For example, patients may struggle to use a comb to comb their hair, and may instead move it around, up and down or even mimic bruising their teeth with the comb. Ideomotor apraxia results from damage to the dominant parietal lobe.

54. F Ideational apraxia

This is a neurological disorder, which explains the loss of the ability to conceptualise, plan, and execute the complex sequence of motor actions involving the use of tools or objects in everyday life.

55. F Primary universal emotions

Ekman and Friesen contributed to the concept of primary universal emotions. All humans express these expressions facially in the same way, which suggests that these are innate. These six emotions are: surprise, fear, disgust, anger, happiness, and sadness.

56. C Hierarchy of needs

According to Maslow, there is a pyramid and hierarchy of needs. Those in the lower part of the pyramid are closely related to innate, physiological needs. The needs of the lower order must be satisfied before it is possible to satisfy higher-order needs. The levels are: self-actualisation, aesthetic, cognitive, self-esteem, belonging/social, safety and lastly physical/physiological.

57. E Learned helplessness

Seligman demonstrated the concept of learned helplessness in his experiments with dogs in which they were strapped and given a series of shocks. The dogs learned that no behaviour on their part had any effect on whether they did or did not receive the shock. He later tried to explain depression in humans in terms of learned helplessness.

58. D Broca's area

This is the major speech area, which occupies Broca's areas 44 and 45, i.e. opercular and triangular zones of the inferior frontal gyrus.

59. H Wernicke's area

This is the sensory speech and language area, occupying Broca's areas 42 and 22, i.e. posterior part of the auditory association cortex of the superior temporal gyrus.

60. A Angular gyrus

This is Broca's area 39, which has connections with the somatosensory, visual and auditory association cortices.

61. B, C Concept-based community. Democratic analytic community

Therapeutic community is applied to a wide range of institutions. These are based on two different types of historical concepts that emerged from two specific therapeutic communities. They were the democratic–analytic community and the community-based community.

62. D, G Democratisation. Reality confrontation

Rappaport described four themes, which emerged as the key values that staff held about treatment. These include: democratisation, permissiveness, communalism and reality confrontation.

63. E, G Humanistic. Psychoanalytic

Transactional analysis is a model of psychotherapy and theory of personality which integrates psychoanalytic concepts with humanistic philosophies.

64. J Treatment contracts

A distinguishing feature of transactional analysis is the use of a formal treatment contract.

65. B, K Games. Transactions

The four cornerstones of transactional analysis theory are: ego states, transactions, games and scripts.

66. D 4

Hippocrates described four temperaments, which include: melancholic, sanguine, phlegmatic and choleric. According to this theory, people with a melancholic temperament are introverted and thoughtful. People with a sanguine temperament are impulsive, pleasure seeking and sociable. People with a phlegmatic temperament are relaxed, quiet, warm and sometimes lazy. People with a choleric temperament are leaders and ambitious.

67. J, K Phlegmatic. Sanguine

Hippocrates described four temperaments, which include: melancholic, sanguine, phlegmatic and choleric. People with a sanguine temperament are considered to be impulsive and the pleasure-seeking type. They are also sociable and emotional. People with a choleric temperament are considered ambitious and leader-like personalities. Those with a melancholic temperament are found to be introverted and thoughtful people. People with a phlegmatic temperament are considered to be relaxed, warm and quiet personalities.

68. H Moral insanity

This term was coined by Prichard in the mid-nineteenth century. Before Prichard, Pinel described the concept of moral insanity. Moral insanity referred to the existence of abnormal emotions and/or behaviours in the absence of intellectual disability or an acute mental illness. The concept of moral insanity was later used in describing psychopathic personality and McNaughton's rule.